Calisthenics for Beginners

Get in Shape and Stay in Shape for the Rest of your Life without Going to the Gym

Daily Calisthenics

© Copyright 2020 - All rights reserved.

The content contained within this book may not be reproduced, duplicated or transmitted without direct written permission from the author or the publisher.

Under no circumstances will any blame or legal responsibility be held against the publisher, or author, for any damages, reparation, or monetary loss due to the information contained within this book, either directly or indirectly.

Legal Notice:

This book is copyright protected. It is only for personal use. You cannot amend, distribute, sell, use, quote or paraphrase any part, or the content within this book, without the consent of the author or publisher.

Disclaimer Notice:

Please note the information contained within this document is for educational and entertainment purposes only. All effort has been executed to present accurate, up to date, reliable, complete information. No warranties of any kind are declared or implied. Readers acknowledge that the author is not engaged in the rendering of legal, financial, medical or professional advice. The content within this book has been derived from various sources. Please consult a licensed professional before attempting any techniques outlined in this book.

By reading this document, the reader agrees that under no circumstances is the author responsible for any losses, direct or indirect, that are incurred as a result of the use of the information contained within this document, including, but not limited to, errors, omissions, or inaccuracies.

Table of Contents

INTRODUCTION 1

   WHY SPECIFICALLY CALISTHENICS 2
      What Do You Stand to Gain? 4
      Questions All Beginners Have 6

CHAPTER 1: MINDSET – WHO IS THIS BOOK FOR? 9

   WHAT IS CALISTHENICS? 9
   HOW YOU BENEFIT FROM CALISTHENICS 11
   HOW TO START WITH CALISTHENICS 13
      Build Foundations: Earn Your Right to Progress 14
      Don't Compare Yourself to Others 15
      Combine Strength with Movement 16
      Trust Your Body 18
      Focus on Core Alignment 19

CHAPTER 2: CALISTHENICS PRINCIPLES 21

   OVERLOAD 22
   SAID PRINCIPLE 24
   PROGRESSIVE OVERLOAD 25
      Leverage Training: Body vs. Machines 27
      Resistance 27
   TOP THREE PROBLEMS AND HOW TO RESOLVE THEM 29
      Freedom 29
      Variety 30
      Simplicity 30
   THE SOLUTIONS TO THESE PROBLEMS 31
   KEY RULES AND FOCAL POINTS 32
      Patience and Consistency 32
      No Cheating 32
      Set Realistic Goals 33
      Stop Comparing Yourself to Others 33

Maintain Diet and Lean Muscle Weight 34
Proper Training Plan 35
Stomp Your Ego Down 35

CHAPTER 3: FLEXIBILITY AND MOBILITY 37

FLEXIBILITY AND MOBILITY EXERCISES 38
OVERHEAD MOBILITY 44

CHAPTER 4: SAFETY, REST, AND RECOVERY 49

SAFETY: HOW TO PREVENT INJURY IN CALISTHENICS 50
CALISTHENICS REST AND RECOVERY 53
HOW TO PLAN CALISTHENICS REST DAYS 56
What are Rest Days? 57

CHAPTER 5: REBALANCE THE SCALES 61

LIFE LESSONS... 62
Discipline 62
Learn to Manage the Fear of Failure 63
Self-Control.. 64
Self-Reliance 64
PHYSICAL BENEFITS 66
Bone Density.. 67
Chronic Conditions... 67
Cognitive Decline 68
Energy Levels 68
Flexibility, Mobility, and Balance..................................... 68
Greater Stamina 68
Immune System 69
Insomnia and Sleep.. 69
Muscle Strength and Tone... 69
Performance of Everyday Tasks....................................... 69
Posture 70
Risk of Injury 70
Self-Esteem 70
Sense of Wellbeing 70
Weight-Management and Muscle to Fat Ratio................ 71
Mental and Emotional Wellbeing.................................... 71
Giving... 71

- *Relating* 72
- *Exercising* 72
- *Appreciating* 72
- *Trying Out* 73
- *Direction* 73
- *Resilience* 74
- HOW TO BALANCE HEALTHY EATING SOCIALLY 75
  - *Check the Menu* 76
  - *Healthy Snack Before Arrival* 76
  - *Water* 77
  - *Check How Food is Prepped and Cooked* 77
  - *Order First* 77
  - *Double Up on Appetizers* 77
  - *Mindful Eating* 78
  - *Eat Slowly and Chew Well* 78
  - *Coffee Instead of Dessert* 78
  - *Request a Healthy Swap* 79
  - *Dressings and Sauces on the Side* 79
  - *Bread Basket* 79
  - *Salad or Soup Starters* 80
  - *Share or Go Half-Portion* 80
  - *Alcohol, Mixers, and Sweetened Drinks* 80
  - *Tomato-Based vs. Creamy Sauces* 81
  - *Be Wary of Health Claims* 81

CHAPTER 6: THE FUEL FOR LEAN LIVING 83

- GENERAL DIET RECOMMENDATIONS 86
- DIET PLAN IDEAS 88
- EATING TIPS AND MEAL IDEAS 94
  - *Breakfast* 95
  - *Lunch and Dinner* 100

CHAPTER 7: GETTING STARTED WITH SMOOTHIES 105

- *Frozen Fruit vs. Fresh* 106
- *Make-Ahead Smoothie Packs* 106
- *Quick Fix Remedies* 107
- *Substitutions* 110
- *Blending Tips and Tricks* 114

SMOOTHIE RECIPES 115
   Orange and Mango Recovery Smoothie 115
   Green Breakfast Protein Smoothie 117
   Cinnamon, Oats, and Apple 118
   Acai Berry and Mint 120
   Avocado and Matcha with Vanilla 121
   Cranberry, Banana, and Peanut Butter 123
   Quinoa with Strawberry and Banana 125
   Banana, Peach, and Honey 126
   Pineapple and Raspberries 127
   Cantaloupe and Ginger Smoothie 129

CHAPTER 8: 7-DAY TRAINING GUIDE PLAN 131

MONDAY 131
TUESDAY: BASIC EXERCISES 134
WEDNESDAY: REST 136
THURSDAY 137
FRIDAY: FAT LOSS 139
SATURDAY: CARDIO 140
SUNDAY: REST 140

CHAPTER 9: CALISTHENICS WORKOUT: MUSCLE GROUPS AND BODY SPLITS 141

HOW MUCH SHOULD YOU EXERCISE? 144
HOW TO TRAIN DIFFERENT MUSCLE GROUPS? 145
WHAT IS HYPERTROPHY, AND HOW TO ACHIEVE IT? 149
HOW TO SCHEDULE YOUR WORKOUT SESSIONS 150
   How to Include Cardio Exercises 151
   How to Exercise Your Core 152

CHAPTER 10: 10 TIPS FOR MAKING MOTIVATION LAST 155

WHY HAVE YOU LOST THE MOTIVATION TO EXERCISE? 155
WHEN YOU FEEL LIKE GIVING UP, REMEMBER TO 157
   Start Small 157
   Stick to the Basics 158
   Focus on Consistency Over Intensity 158
   Remember Why You Started 159
   Don't Take an All-Or-Nothing Approach 159

Stick to the Basics *160*
Remind Yourself What's at Stake *160*
Make it Fun! *161*
How to Avoid Future Mistakes 163
Hating on Fat *164*
Poor Diet and Cardio Optimization *164*
Focused on Result, Not the Process *164*

CHAPTER 11: HOW TO TRACK YOUR PROGRESS 167

Intuitive vs Planned Training 168
How to Plan Your Calisthenics Training 170
How to Track Your Progress 173
How to Evaluate Your Progress with Calisthenics 176

CHAPTER 12: 11 BIGGEST MYTHS ABOUT CALISTHENICS 179

Myth #1: The Best Workout Time is Early Morning 180
Always Do Cardio First *181*
Minimum of 20 Minutes Cardio *181*
More Cardio, More Weight Loss *182*
Cardio Machines Record Calories Burnt Accurately *183*
Myth # 2: Crunches and Sit-Ups Equal 6-Pack Abs 183
Myth # 3: Crunches for Core Strength 184
Fat Is Able to Become Muscle, and Vice Versa *184*
Muscle Loss Starts After 7 Days of Being Inactive *184*
Myth #4: No Pain, No Gain 185
Myth #5: Running Is Better Than Walking 185
Myth #6: Sports Drinks Are Healthy 186
Myth #7: Treadmills and Running Outdoors Are Equal 186
Myth #8: Exercise Makes You Hungry 187
Never Do Workouts on an Empty Stomach *187*
Myth #9: Toning My Muscles Is All I Need to Do 187
Myth #10: Men and Women Cannot Do the Same Workouts 188
Women Should Lift Lighter and Do More Reps *188*
Yoga Is Not Proper Exercise *189*
Myth #11: Stretching Is A Must to Prevent Injuries 189

CONCLUSION 191

REFERENCES 199

BEFORE YOU START READING! I have this special bonus that I am going to reveal to you:

https://bit.ly/DailyJayyy

Up there is a link that will direct you to a website where you can get a fitness calculator. I actually used this exact same calculator to get an estimate and track how many calories I needed to eat in a day to achieve the body of my dreams when I was just getting started in my journey.

Just insert your name and email and it will be sent straight to your email.

Introduction

"Taking care of your body, no matter what your age, is an investment."

-Oprah Winfrey

These simple words, spoken by Oprah Winfrey, are profound and wise. It is never too late to start taking care of your body. Whatever effort you put in is a huge investment with incredible returns. You improve your overall looks, your health, your quality of life, and your relationships with everyone you interact with. Maintaining your body completely changes how you look at the world. Your mindset changes, and you see the positive in situations where before you saw only the negative.

The goal of this book is to provide you with the necessary tools to begin calisthenics with confidence, backed up by facts and not people's opinions. This book will show you that you can have the body you have always wanted, without spending hours in the gym each day, nor spending a fortune on exercise machines and equipment.

The world is currently experiencing a pandemic that impacts every human on the planet. If we learn only one thing from this, it is that we must face the critical importance of taking care of our bodies even when we are unable to go to the gym or participate in the sports we love. This is the goal of this book, to show you that it can be done, and how to do it.

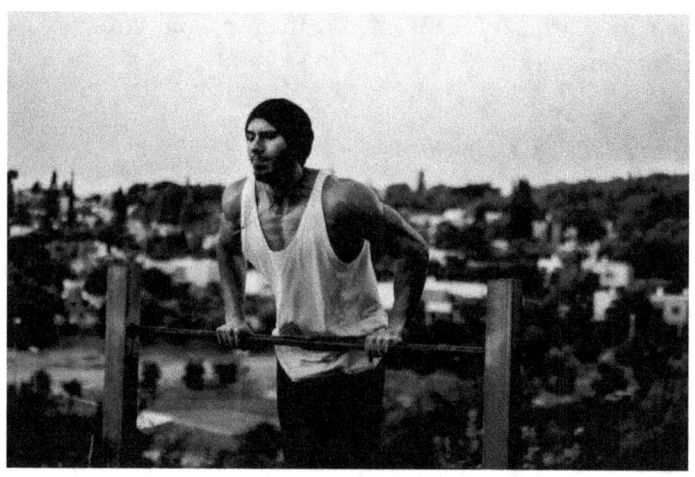

Why Specifically Calisthenics

Calisthenics is not only for super fit athletes who wish to maintain their ripped looks and fitness levels. It is accessible to the majority of people of different ages, fitness levels, and different states of health. Today there are specially developed calisthenics routines for seniors as well as school-going children, and it places no limitations on gender.

In 2017, the Sport and Exercise Sciences Research Unit at the University of Palermo, Italy published the results of a study called 'The effects of a calisthenics training intervention on posture, strength, and body composition." The study concluded that calisthenics training is a "feasible and effective training solution to improve posture, strength, and body composition without the use of any major training equipment".

Calisthenics differs from other forms of exercise and appeals to people for many reasons, such as the following:

- Anyone who is out of shape and wants to change how they feel and look can do calisthenics.

- You can do this form of exercise literally anywhere and at any time. You are not bound to a specific place or time frame.

- People who experience health problems and want to change to a healthier lifestyle can do calisthenics.

- Anyone who does not like going to gyms and working out on all the machines available there will enjoy calisthenics.

- Every person who prefers their workout routines to be natural and free, and not dependent on any specific piece of equipment, without which they would be unable to exercise, will prefer calisthenics.

- People who want to use their own body weight to increase their strength, muscle tone, and development can use calisthenics.

- Anyone who has fallen into a rut with their current training program of monotonous exercise workouts will like calisthenics.

What Do You Stand to Gain?

Calisthenics brings literally endless gains into your life, and we will go into detail about the specific benefits in Chapter 5. The gains calisthenics will bring you fall into four broad categories that each cover a very wide range of benefits.

Endurance

Consistently practicing calisthenics routines builds your muscular endurance, and over time will build up your body's resistance to muscular fatigue. As you progress with calisthenics, you will keep challenging your body until you involve the muscles throughout your entire body in building endurance. The muscular endurance of your cardiovascular system also builds through calisthenics routines, which is a huge health benefit for anyone.

Strength

Calisthenics is associated with building muscle strength, which it does incredibly well. Often, however, people do not realize how much calisthenics also strengthens your joints and contributes to bone health. This is exactly why the US Military uses calisthenics in their basic training for the building of strength, and also to help prevent injuries. Using calisthenics for building muscular strength is much gentler than, for instance, weight lifting, which takes a toll on the body with greater wear and tear.

Flexibility

When you start out with calisthenics, you become acutely aware of stiffness and tightness in body parts you always considered to be very flexible. This is where the benefits of calisthenics workouts really kick in, as these exercises have the full range of movements that your body should be capable of. The longer you do calisthenics, the more flexible your entire body becomes as your strength increases and your body adapts.

Changes to the Metabolic Rate

Calisthenics strength training builds muscle mass, and at the same time tones every part of your body. This means that your resting metabolic rate will be higher than before. Thus, your body continues to burn more calories during the resting phase and throughout your entire day. The second way your metabolic rate changes is that when you consistently do calisthenics workouts, your heart rate rises. This represents aerobic exercises. Aerobics is recognized by doctors worldwide as one of the most effective ways for the human body to burn calories. Calisthenics, therefore, addresses the problem of burning excess fat and calories from two directions, by changing your metabolic rate to work more effectively.

Questions All Beginners Have

It is natural for beginners to have questions and uncertainties when they are about to embark not only on a new exercise regime, but in reality, on a major change in lifestyle and mindset.

This book tackles the important questions and provides insightful answers and guidance for questions such as the following:

- Is there a greater risk of injuries without gym staff to assist and guide me?

- Will calisthenics definitely be able to address my personal goal or issue?

- Will I be able to see results quickly?

- How will I stay motivated in the long term?

- Does science back up the principles of calisthenics?

- What equipment will I need to buy?

- Will I keep on seeing results after the initial changes?

- What benefits will I gain from doing calisthenics?

- What are the dos and don'ts of calisthenics training?

- Is there an average amount of weight that can be lost through practicing calisthenics?

- What are the common mistakes people make?

Chapter 1:

Mindset – Who Is This Book for?

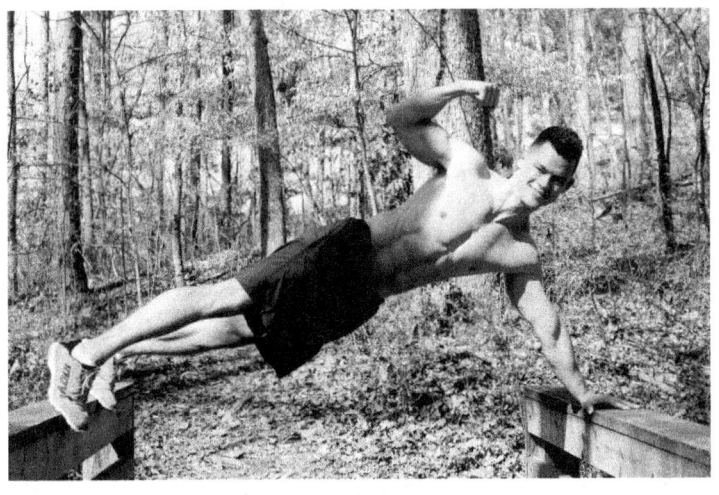

What is Calisthenics?

Calisthenics is a type of exercise that uses the body's own weight to gain strength. It improves your muscular volume and shapes your body for proper athletic form, depending on your own natural features and tendencies. Calisthenics is a fitness form that uses body weight and gravity to build strength and promote health. The term originated from the Greek words "Kalos" and "Stenos", the first word meaning beauty, and the second meaning strength (Thomas et. al., 2017). Aside from bodybuilding, it's commonly used with school children, in gymnastics, and in outdoor practicing.

One of the famous calisthenics exercisers is Hannibal Lanham (Hannibal for King), who attracted the attention of millions to this discipline by showing his skills in parks in Queens, New York.

Kenneth Gallarzo, the co-founder of the World Calisthenics Organization (WCO), started off as a fitness trainer. He became interested in calisthenics after seeing another person in the gym doing a fascinating exercise he had never seen before. After researching calisthenics, Gallarzo came to understand that this form of exercise is a great foundation for other strength-gaining disciplines.

However, calisthenics is more than just another commercial exercise program that promises a lot and delivers little. Studies showed that calisthenics effectively improves body composition, strength, and posture (Thomas et. al., 2017). The recorded benefits of calisthenics are numerous, and will be explained in more detail as we go.

How You Benefit from Calisthenics

Your body isn't made to only move forwards and backwards. Calisthenics adds rotations, twists, pushes, pulls, squats, and jumps to your movement. Calisthenics exercises require more muscle use for you to build muscle when done at a moderate and slow rate, and more calorie burning when done at a slower rate with more cardio training. This is because higher muscle engagement also increases fat burning. Practicing calisthenics will help you become stronger, fitter, and slimmer. Aside from this, there are more proven benefits of these exercises:

- **Flexibility.** As you don't need equipment for calisthenics, you can exercise anywhere and anytime. You don't have to commit to a certain schedule or make the time to go to the gym, which is great if you're busy, or if having a constant schedule (although recommended) is challenging for you. Instead, you should dedicate a space for freestyle training, like a functional frame or Swedish ladders. As you can see, the only commitment with calisthenics is to plan well and actually do the exercises with discipline the right way.

- **Naturally toned shape.** Calisthenics will help you burn fat, increase your power and strength, and strengthen your entire body. It will boost the secretion of endorphins and help you feel more energized. Calisthenics trains multiple groups of muscles at the same time. For example, push-ups train the spine, abdominal muscles, chest, and arms. This way, your body will look more proportionate, and you won't worry about balancing your exercises. Your body will shape and sculpt in a natural way that fits your shape and body type, with muscles being toned to their optimum level.

- **Mindset change.** Calisthenics helps you connect with your body and improve physical awareness. Repetitive workouts can become boring, so exercisers lose motivation. However, calisthenics, while including repetitions, changes its types of exercises and exercise routines. Once you master one skill level, you will move on to the next one. Your challenges increase as your body shapes up.

- Last, but not least, calisthenics prevents physical injury while exercising. This is because the exercises don't allow you to overstrain a certain muscle type.

Calisthenics sound much more appealing with the idea of not having to pay for a gym membership, pump iron, and schedule around your weekly workouts. At the same time, doing exercises that shape your body naturally is healthier and has greater psychological and health benefits than pumping iron.

How to Start with Calisthenics

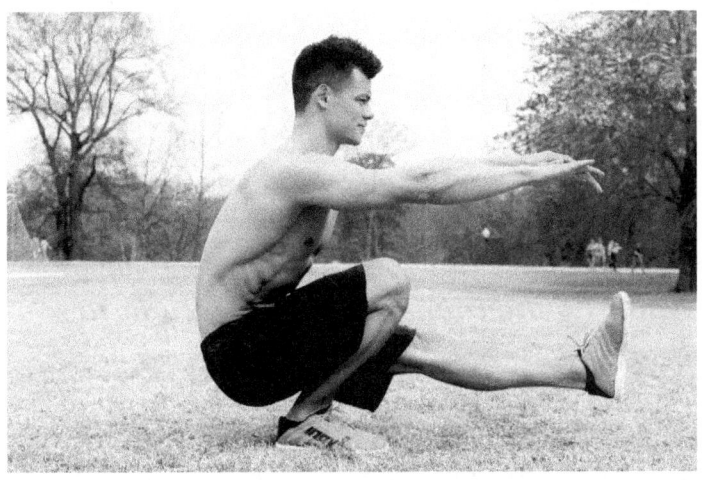

So, how should you begin? The following sections will discuss some of the basic principles of calisthenics and the bare essentials you need for a successful body transformation.

Calisthenics is all about exploring your natural potential and pushing boundaries further and further, in a way suitable to your individual body type and shape. Surpassing one level after the other will eventually give you superb strength, and will become a fun way to exercise. Bodyweight training with calisthenics is often difficult to start. Not knowing things like where and how to exercise and how to get going can be frustrating, but a proper mindset and knowledge of exercise routines should help you start.

As you decide to start with calisthenics, you'll probably be confused about how to start correctly. Should you simply do more planks and pushups? Or is there a bit more to organizing your workouts for the best result? The rule of thumb is that most beginners make some mistakes, but they are easy to correct. Exercises are learned with practice, and results become more visible the more you exercise. To start, focus on building a proper mindset for learning and practicing calisthenics.

Build Foundations: Earn Your Right to Progress

Earning your right to progress means first building foundations for long-term exercise. Most people who are just starting with calisthenics get addicted to the initial progress. You're trying new routines and getting better by the day. Your brain and body are being stimulated, and you naturally want to go further and further. Still, it is important to stay focused on your body and have a clear direction to follow. Upscaling will start to become challenging at one point or another, and unless you're ready to confront these roadblocks, your motivation might suffer.

So, how do you start with calisthenics? Although you probably got to know this concept by seeing exercisers doing advanced movements, as a beginner, you'll have to start slowly, for the sake of both your health and safety. Ideally, you'll start with basic exercises like:

- **Press-up.** This exercise can be adjusted for beginners. To do a beginner press-up, do press-ups with your hands on a bench and feet on the ground. Once you master this exercise, you can move on to regular press-ups. For starters, do up to 20 repetitions.

- **Dips.** After you're able to do 20 press-ups, you can start exercising with dips. To perform a dip, pull yourself up on a bar and bend your elbows to dip down, then straighten back up.

- Squats, lunges, and planks.

- **Rows.** This is an interesting exercise where you hold onto a bar, facing toward your chest, and lean backward, with feet firmly on the ground. You should make sure that your back is as parallel with the floor as possible.

Don't Compare Yourself to Others

The second rule is to never compare yourself with others. Comparing yourself to those who started before you and have a long background with calisthenics can ruin your motivation. Every person progresses at their own pace and in their own time. On top of that, everyone's body is different. Your age, health, training history, and how athletic you are now will determine your beginner stage and your direction with exercise. Instead of comparing other people's journey's with your own, be inspired by them and use their progress as motivation for where you want to be.

Combine Strength with Movement

The balance between strength and movement is the key to building natural, lasting strength and vitality. Most people focus only on strength, as it is the most popular goal to pursue. However, as you'll learn, the manifestation of your strength and what you're able to do with it doesn't only rely on your muscles. Instead, balance, flexibility, coordination, and mental clarity gained through balanced exercise will improve both your looks and physical performance. The balance between movement and strength gives you flexibility and mobility in your joints. For starters, if you're having problems with range of motion, which is often the case with those who live a sedentary lifestyle, the following overhead positions will help you improve:

- **Handstands.** Handstands are an exercise that increases body control and strength. Unless you have a background in fitness, you'll only be able to do them once you've set a basis with regular beginner exercises. Notably, risk from injury while attempting handstands as a beginner is low, and your hands won't be able to support your body unless your current physical ability allows it. There are many variations of this exercise, and beginners are best off with the so-called "line handstand", in which you keep your body in a straight line. This position will open your shoulders, strengthen and tighten your core, and protect your back. Long-term, this exercise will help you build skills that are beneficial for other exercises.

- **Human flags.** Feel like turning yourself into a human flag? The good news is that you'll have a fun time doing it, even if you fail. While this exercise also isn't the most beginner-friendly, attempting a beginner version is sure to get your blood running, which is always a good thing. Before you start training to perform a human flag, you will have to be able to hold a single arm hang for 30 seconds, do four sets of 10 pull-ups, and hold a side plank for 45 seconds. This is the very basis of the training, after which you'll train by doing elbow side planks, reach side planks, inclined side planks (five sets of 45 seconds on each side), hanging hip hikers, and pike shoulder push-ups (15-20 repetitions for a half-minute).

Trust Your Body

Given that calisthenics exercises use only the strength and movement of your body, your brain will prevent you from injuring yourself by limiting the movements that are overstraining. You won't be able to use the muscles that are too tight, nor make movements that are too much for your joints to handle, helping you prevent injury and learn how to listen to your body. Moving according to your own body characteristics and possibilities helps you create a more beautiful shape and use your strength, instead of restricting it.

Working with your bodyweight is both one of the biggest advantages and one of the greatest challenges of calisthenics. However, it takes some time to understand how the body adapts and grows from creating resistance on its own. With calisthenics, your body becomes its own weight. As it grows and increases in weight, so does the resistance. As you can see, this is a never-ending process with endless possibilities to advance.

Developing calisthenics skills will require taking good care of your joints. They will be more strained as you exercise harder. Range of motion and the strain put on your connective tissues will increase as you start developing your calisthenics skills. For example, when you do pushups with your initial weight, you'll be working with an easier load, compared to increased body weight after some time spent growing your muscles. This will put extra strain on your joints, but they'll take longer to adapt to this change. This is because your ligaments and tendons don't get the same amount of blood flow as your muscles.

Focus on Core Alignment

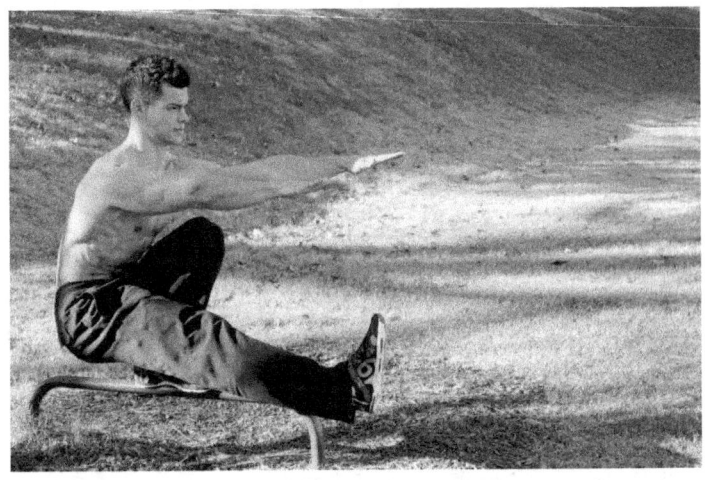

Traditional workouts use machines and other equipment, but calisthenics requires proper body alignment to support your body weight, and for the biggest benefits. Focusing on body alignment requires working your core every time you exercise. To use your core correctly, you should follow the rules that will be explained further in the book to control your body alignment.

Your shoulders give the biggest motion range and allow different movements. However, their stability needs improvement through consistent exercise. Shoulder exercises should be one of your biggest priorities. Shoulder setting and pushing, as well as pulling will be important. Practicing opposing motions helps stabilize your motions.

Balancing your hands is another important aspect of calisthenics. For this, you should practice frog stands in the beginning, and then move on to tiger bends, handstands, elbow levers, and other more challenging exercises.

At the end of the day, your journey should be fun and inspiring. Boredom is a sign that you should switch routines and include new, more challenging exercises. You've now learned what calisthenics is all about, and what you need to do before you start training. But wait! It's not yet time to start doing any exercises. There's still a lot for you to learn for a well-planned, methodical exercise regimen and diet that will produce healthy, visible results. The next chapter will shed more light on calisthenics principles to follow for healthy and safe exercise.

Chapter 2:

Calisthenics Principles

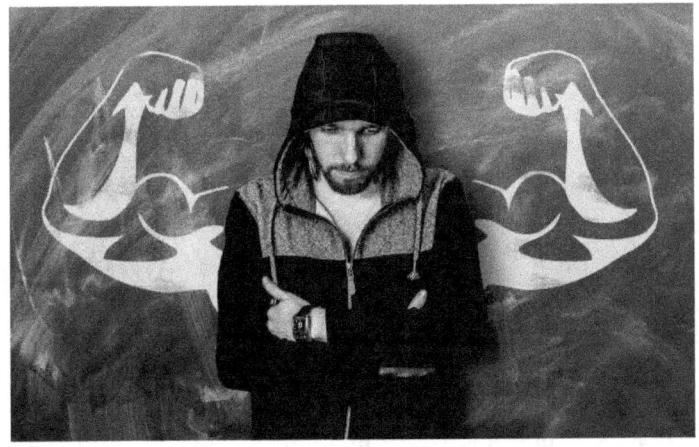

Now that you know what calisthenics is and the advantages over weight lifting, we will discuss calisthenics principles in more detail. Principles in calisthenics show you how to arrange your workouts and specific exercises to get to the best result, and also how to overcome some of the challenges of this training concept. There are numerous exercise programs out there, each designed to produce maximum results for different groups and types of exercisers. However, for any training program to work, one must acknowledge the individual characteristics of each person. Your exercise program will depend on your individual goals and body characteristics. For example, if you want to increase strength, you'll have a different exercise program than if you worked to increase muscle definition. All of this is also affected by your health and previous experience with training, and also by how much time you can devote to exercise. Following general principles when exercising will help you design a more effective exercise program and achieve better results.

When you embrace calisthenics, your whole lifestyle changes. As with any changes, you need to build on strong foundations for success and sustainability in the long run. Calisthenics is not just exercising; it becomes a way of life.

In this chapter, we will go through the key or foundational principles of calisthenics. We will define the most common terminology, specific problems everyone who practices calisthenics faces, and how to resolve it. We will also work through the basic rules and focal points each beginner needs to know and understand. The three basic principles of exercise that apply to anyone, regardless of their skill level, include:

Overload

This principle states that adaptation will happen when your body is exposed to more strain or stress than normal. When you overload your body with higher performance and increased physical strain, it will improve its performance to meet these demands. In this sense, overload is a stimulus, and a much-needed one to see results when exercising. Without it, you'd only see mild to moderate improvements. Your body will adapt to stresses put upon it to handle it better every time, meaning it will make your muscles bigger and bigger. These changes are even visible on a cellular level, with improved cardiovascular performance in those who exercise frequently and intensely. This is how your levels of physical fitness increase, which manifests in faster and better physical performance, and bigger, stronger, better-defined muscles. Below is how you can manipulate overload to generate desired results.

How often do you exercise? Frequency introduces regularity to your exercise program. The rule of thumb is that periods of exercise are followed by periods of recovery. It balances the stress out, and allows your body to heal from the strain and adapt to the new circumstances, which is vital if you want to see any results. Periods of training should be followed by periods of recovery for you to see results, and both of these are essential. Both training and recovery require adequate nutrition and quality sleep. While a proper diet supplies enough fuel for exercise, quality sleep helps your body heal and recover.

The intensity of exercise is also important. You will need an optimum balance in the intensity of exercise to generate enough stress and achieve results, but not too much to burn out or injure yourself. The rule is that the intensity increases by either increasing resistance, or increasing the number of repetitions. However, keep in mind that too many repetitions may get in the way of building strength. Instead, you can add exercises, shuffle exercise modes, or change the tempo to increase the intensity of your workouts.

Exercise duration depends on exercise intensity. It's recommended for more intense exercises to be performed for shorter amounts of time, and less intense ones for longer. This will give you enough intensity without overload.

SAID Principle

The SAID principle stands for Specific Adaptation to Imposed Demands. This principle dictates targeting specific goals or activities to improve skills. This principle states that the type of adaptation that will occur from the exercise depends on the type of stress placed upon a particular part of the body, a muscle, or a muscle group. To achieve your goals with exercise, you'll choose the kind of exercises you do based on the result you're trying to achieve. One example of differing results is wanting to become a fast runner, versus wanting to lose weight and improve health. The first goal will be best achieved with outdoor sprinting, while the second will need a focus on cardio exercise, body strength, and lifestyle changes. Simply put, your training sessions should align with your goals.

SAID also means that the human body has the ability to adapt when neurological and biomechanical demands are imposed on it. Thus, you need to work smarter instead of working harder blindly. The SAID principle is your guideline.

- **Specific:** Do not choose your activities randomly. Choose science-based activities that have been proven to work.

- **Adaptation to**: Be very clear about what adaptation you want to happen during this phase of training.

- **Imposed:** Activities must be performed consistently over a specific time frame.

- **Demands:** Perform your chosen activity(s) with sufficient intensity to cause the adaptation you desire, while performing the activity correctly and safely.

Progressive Overload

The principle of progressive overload means that you gradually and continuously increase the demands that you place on your entire musculoskeletal system. Doing this helps you to gain strength, endurance, and muscle size. So, in order to gain strength and develop muscles, you have to keep making your muscles work harder than they did before. So, once your muscles get used to, for example, lifting a specific weight or doing a specific exercise, you will then increase the weight or increase the reps and sets to make your muscles work harder again.

Your exercise will have to become progressively more difficult to achieve harder performance levels. Unless you increase the intensity of exercise progressively, you will reach a plateau. Good results will require progressive overload, and a significant transformation will require long, dedicated work. The basic resistance exercises can be broken down into:

- **Multi-joint exercises**, also known as core exercises, like squats. These exercises will require stabilizing your torso to keep your spine in a neutral position. They are also called structural exercises. A squat, for example, includes stress placed on the spine, and requires engaging core muscles to keep it stabilized. It also engages ankle, hip, and knee joints and puts a strain on the gluteus maximus, quadriceps, and hamstring muscles.

- Core exercises can be further broken down by increasing movement speed. The so-called explosive, or power exercises are done at higher speeds.

- **Single-joint exercises**, or assistance exercises. These exercises engage only one primary joint and recruit either one small or one large muscle group.

Leverage Training: Body vs. Machines

Using your own bodyweight to exercise, instead of machines, is the most natural and practical way to exercise. Body leverage training has become extremely popular because it is so functional, and because you can do it anywhere, at any time, and alone or in a group.

Reps and Sets

Below are the number of reps and sets you need to do during leverage training to fit your specific goals.

- Strength: 5-8 reps
- Power: 2-4 reps
- Endurance: 15-20 reps
- Hypertrophy: 8-12 reps

Resistance

Resistance exercises mean that you use an external form of resistance to contract your muscles for toning, strengthening, building mass, and endurance training. The great part is that you do not need gym machines to achieve this with calisthenics. You can use your own body weight or a set of resistance bands, or even grab a few tins of food off the pantry shelf. Basically, anything that is handy to make your muscles contract will work.

Good examples of calisthenics resistance training tools are:

- **Resistance bands.** These provide great resistance when stretched, for example, around arms or legs.

- **Any form of suspension equipment.** Suspension bars and rings, or even a sturdy tree branch will do. The suspension uses your own body weight and gravity to perform the exercises.

- **Free weights**, with the classical equipment for strength training being kettlebells, dumbbells, and barbells, but a couple of sandbags work just as well.

- **Medicine balls** are used to great effect for resistance training and are suitable for all ages and levels of fitness.

- **Bodyweight only**. Getting into shape and building a great physique does not depend on a gym and all the machines lined up there. All it really takes is you using your own body weight and perseverance. You can do chin-ups, squats, and push-ups anywhere and anytime, and you don't need a gym membership for this. Bodyweight resistance training works great when you travel, whether for work or for fun, and you don't need to drag bags full of bulky equipment around with you.

Top Three Problems and How to Resolve Them

All beginners face three problems, or drawbacks, when they start their calisthenics journey. That said, it is not the end of the world, as the answer is to take the problems on board, then find the solution and implement it.

Freedom

Yes, it does sound strange, but the freedom that calisthenics gives people is also a drawback. You are not bound to be at the gym and you can do your workout anywhere. You are also not bound by a time schedule and you are not booking time on equipment. For some people, this is not good because they struggle without a specific routine. This could lead to inconsistency in doing their workouts regularly. The other end of the scale is also a possibility, as you can work out literally anywhere and anytime, so you might fall into the trap of doing too much, too often.

Variety

The saying that variety is the spice of life is truly correct. For example, there are 21 different ways to do push-ups, and if you are only familiar with two or three ways to do them, your workout routines will become boring. It is important to bring variety into your workouts because once boredom sets in, it could lead to demotivation.

Here again, you could be at the other end of the scale, where you want to try every possible variation of each exercise. This means you are not focusing on any single type of exercise, but randomly working out. This will negatively impact the path you wish your progression to follow. Yes, it can be confusing for beginners, but as with everything in life, you must find a good balance to keep you motivated and on the path you chose.

Simplicity

The very simplicity of calisthenics can be a drawback for some people. They find it difficult to deal with plateaus that might last for a long while, or they become bored with following a set workout plan. Others feel that, unless they use tools and equipment, they are not making noticeable progress. Should you find that you are getting bored, it is time to make some changes to your workout plan.

The Solutions to These Problems

To resolve the above problems, you need to come up with a disciplined and strict workout plan to keep you focused and always pushing forward.

Create a workout routine from where you are now, with the focus on where you want to be.

Work out a plan on paper or on your computer, and print it out. It is important to have a visual reminder of what your goals are and which exercise routines will push you to achieve those goals.

Make sure that you include your workout session in your daily calendar, at a convenient time for you.

These actions will sharpen your focus and also prevent you from doing too much or too little.

Key Rules and Focal Points

Throughout this book, we will repeat this: calisthenics is more than just physical exercises. It is a mind and body experience. As you master your own body, your mind plays a very large part in this for you, in order to reap all the benefits of calisthenics. It is therefore very important to bring your mind and body into balance when you start out with calisthenics.

Patience and Consistency

Most people do not have an overabundance of patience in whatever they do. They want to get it done and see the results ASAP. Two words each beginner must keep in mind at all times are patience and consistency. Without cultivating patience in your workouts and working hard, you will not achieve the results you strive for. Your workouts will become inconsistent when you want instant results, as you will become despondent. The key is patience and keeping at it.

No Cheating

There are no quick fixes and shortcuts when you do your workouts. Your body is an incredible biological machine designed to do an amazing range of different forms of motion. To achieve your goals and reap the lifelong benefits of calisthenics, you need to focus on doing the full range of motion that your body is capable of. Cheating and trying to take shortcuts is futile; you are only cheating yourself. Focus on doing each exercise to perfection, and do this every time you do a workout. Don't cheat yourself. You are worth putting in the full effort every time.

Set Realistic Goals

When you start out with calisthenics, everything is new, and you see improvements with every workout. This is a very exciting time, and you have all the right to enjoy this. Over time, though, as your body becomes fitter and stronger, your rate of improvement will slow down. This is natural, and to avoid disappointment you need to set realistic goals of what you want to achieve in a logically achievable workout plan.

Stop Comparing Yourself to Others

As a beginner, you will be doing generalized workouts. This is how it should be. Through generalization, you learn and find out whether you want to progress to be a specialist. For example, you might pick a focus and specialize in handstand routines. Do not compare yourself to anyone, especially not anyone who has been doing calisthenics for a long time and who specializes in it, because you put undue pressure on yourself. As a generalist, you'll do a large variety of workouts, whereas a specialist only focuses on his or her specialty. Your progress will be slower because your focus is much wider, and this is normal and nothing to worry about.

Use social media logically to get more information and ideas. Do not compare yourself to the celebrities posting and boasting about their progress and their achievements. Yes, acknowledge that these people work hard to achieve their personal goals, because that is true, but do not use them as the yardstick for your own progress. Social media often does much more harm to beginners, and even to more experienced practitioners of calisthenics. The whole celebrity hype can erode people's self-worth. Your goal with calisthenics is to be the best you possible, not strive to be a copy of anyone else.

Maintain Diet and Lean Muscle Weight

Your diet plays a huge role in your progress with calisthenics. You cannot bulk up through eating junk food, or just enormous quantities of food. It simply does not work this way. You have to strive to achieve and maintain lean muscle weight through a good training program and a balanced diet. Fat body weight cannot replace lean muscle weight. Your food intake and your training program must be in line with the specific objectives you want to achieve.

Proper Training Plan

You must have a properly set up training program worked out for your specific needs and goals. You cannot just stumble along doing random exercises and expect to gain any benefits. Without a training program, you will fall into the trap of just doing what is easiest to do and what comes to mind. You will then do whatever you feel like doing in your daily workout sessions, instead of what you need to do to achieve your goal. Grabbing random exercises for your training will lead to random progress that takes you nowhere.

Create a training program and stick with it for a minimum of 6 weeks before reevaluating your goals. You can then decide whether you wish to continue longer with this specific training program, or move on to another one.

Stomp Your Ego Down

Ego has no place in any form of physical training, and this definitely is the case with calisthenics. This goes for men and women. You cannot allow your ego to rule you. All you will achieve is getting injured. This will set your training back and make it more difficult to achieve your goals. Learn from the countless people who have allowed their egos to short circuit their logic. Stomp your ego flat into the dust and do calisthenics the right way, without overreaching yourself.

Chapter 3:

Flexibility and Mobility

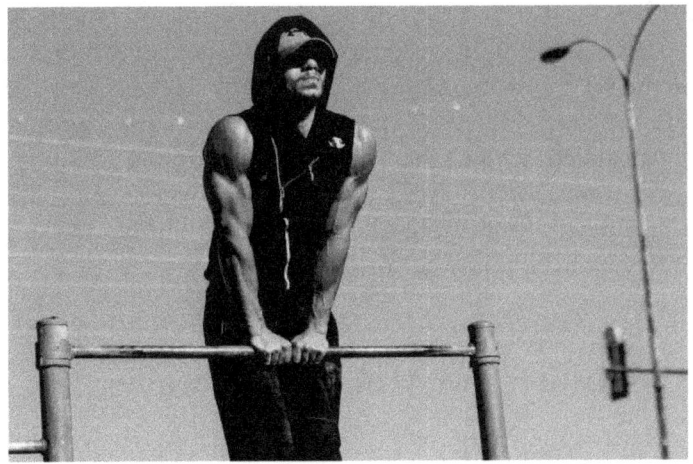

Flexibility and mobility are often overlooked in fitness. Diet, muscle strength, definition, weight loss, and other training aspects tend to prevail over paying attention to the mobility of your joints and tendons. However, flexibility and mobility have far greater importance than most people realize. They reduce pain during daily activities, and are important for cardiovascular health. Many suffer from chronic lower back pain, which is caused by the lack of flexibility and mobility in the body, as well as tight hamstrings.

A sedentary lifestyle causes the lower back to become rounded, which affects body weight pressure on the lower back and causes pain. The lack of mobility in your lower back links with reduced productivity and diminished work performance as well.

Studies also found that flexibility is linked to mortality. The less flexible people are, the higher the chance of cardiovascular disease. Both flexibility and mobility refer to the ability of your joints to move through a range of motion. Mobility can also reduce due to tightness in muscles, which doesn't allow proper physical activity and increases the risk of injury. Studies also found that flexibility and mobility exercises should be used as a preventive measure against injury, and not only when the injury occurs.

Flexibility and Mobility Exercises

Working on your mobility will help prevent injuries and increase strength. As a beginner in calisthenics, you're most likely focused on the number of exercises you can do and the repetitions that will create the desired result. While this is understandable, long-term strength and balance require exercising mobility and flexibility. Mobility includes two different aspects of flexibility:

- **Passive flexibility**: Low-stress muscle, tendon, and ligament flexibility, like doing splits on the ground.

- **Dynamic flexibility**: high-stress flexibility in your ligaments, tendons, and muscles. Exercising dynamic flexibility is important to improve fitness ability levels and maintain flexibility under high stress. This requires a high level of strength, as well as exercising ligament and tendon flexibility. Simply put, muscles shouldn't be your only point of focus when exercising. Your tendons and ligaments require the same amount of attention, as they suffer an equal amount of stress when you're exercising, but take longer to recover and adapt.

Regardless of your muscle strength, you can get injured doing mundane daily tasks if your ligaments aren't flexible enough. Poor motility can be corrected with certain stretching exercises designed to improve your flexibility. Although they might appear boring because they don't improve strength and grow muscles, they're necessary for you to stay healthy in the long run. Working with your bodyweight helps this, because your body has an instinct to balance itself and, as said earlier, won't allow you to make movements that will injure it. But what can you do to improve mobility? There are a couple of types of exercises that you can do:

- **Passive stretching**. Shoulder extension exercises include back levers, V sits, and skin the cats. They stretch tight muscles in your shoulders and hands, particularly in your biceps, that get in the way of extending shoulders properly. They will help extend muscles in the backs of your arms and help exercises using weights.

- **Passive shoulder stretches.** Doing exercises with tight shoulders can not only reduce their efficiency, but also lead to tearing muscles and rupturing tendons. Exercises like V sits and German hangs, particularly their advanced versions, will require a lot of shoulder flexibility.

What should your stretches look like? You should start slowly with three sets of one-minute holds, three times each week. After you gain more experience and mobility, you should focus on doing more German hangs (skinning the cat), starting with up to five sets of half-minute holds. Once you've mastered beginner stretches, you can move on to do more demanding warm-up exercises, such as:

- **Motion range exercises.** These exercises take joints through full-range motions. The tension doesn't have to be high with these exercises, but they're still essential. These exercises include mobility exercises for shoulders, including the one described below.

- **Shoulder dislocates.** These exercises are simple, and can greatly improve the mobility of your shoulders. To do them, you'll need a wide grip on a light bar or a dowel rod. With arms raised in front of you and extended elbows, maneuver the bar as high and behind your head as possible. The rod should weigh between five and ten pounds. If lighter, the exercise becomes about passive flexibility. Here, you want to engage muscles as well, not just joints and ligaments. As a beginner, you should start with a wider grip and bring your hands closer together as you progress. When you're able to do the exercise with hands only slightly apart from shoulders, you can increase the weight of the rod and go back to exercising the wide grip again. Your mobility will increase as you increase the challenge, and progression will always be done by increasing weight and starting over.

The main focus of this exercise is for you to achieve a full shoulder blade, or scapula, range of motion. Your scapula should protract with your arms extended outwards, and your shoulder blades should stretch. Then, they should retract as you lift your hands and pull them behind your head. Shoulder dislocates aren't speed exercises, and should be done slowly and patiently.

- **Skinning the cats.** Not literally, of course. This exercise mimics the position of the animal in said situation, and it's far less grueling and difficult than it sounds. It's done by hanging from a pull-up bar and raising the body up and in front of you. You should practice doing the movement as far out as possible, then slowly getting back to the start position. The first couple of repetitions might be slow and difficult if you're a beginner, but that's not a problem. This exercise engages both a lot of strength and a lot of flexibility, and you should be patient with yourself before you're able to produce Instagram-worthy repetitions. Your ability will improve as you repeat the exercise. To practice safely, your shoulder blades should be slightly retracted when you're hanging from the bar, and before you've started the movement. Doing so will help you lift your body more easily to start the movement.

- **Shoulder distractions.** This exercise doesn't bring your shoulders to their full motion range. It stretches ligaments, as it distracts your upper arm bone from your joint capsule. The exercise feels pleasant even with an injury. To do it, you should use a five-to-ten-pound weight and bend over. Rest the non-swinging hand on a chair, and then relax and swing the other arm in a circular motion, both clockwise and counterclockwise. When you do this exercise, synovial fluid lubricates the joint and helps it become more flexible. However, it should be done slowly and patiently. Don't rush to speed or to use a full motion range. The purpose of the exercise is to distract the humerus, improving ligament mobility in your shoulders as a result. There's never too much of this exercise. Ideally, you'll do it every day, and as often as you like.

Mobility exercises are a great warm-up before doing handstands, and should be done in two-minute intervals.

Lacking flexibility can not only limit your movement, but also make you feel stiff and slow. Regardless of strength, a lack of flexibility can become limiting to your performance and even everyday activities. Once you've set a strong foundation with push-ups, pull-ups, and dips, more progression will require more flexibility and mobility. Harder exercises, like the back lever, muscle-up, and L-sits will require adding flexibility exercises to your daily routine. These stretching exercises will make it much easier to practice more advanced moves, for example:

- **Better Front Fold exercises.** These stretches help make handstands, hanging leg raises, V-sits, and L-sits easier. These exercises might look as if they only engage the core, but that's not true at all. They also require posterior chain mobility. Foot folds allow you to fight gravity without adding resistance to your muscles. Tight feet and hamstrings are typically present in beginners, and straightening legs during an L-sit appears impossible, regardless of strength. Muscle strength alone won't secure proper V- and L-sits without flexibility exercises. However, once you focus on exercising your hamstrings and the flexibility of your front fold, the resistance in these areas will reduce. To do these exercises correctly, you should try straightening your legs in a comfortable pike position on the floor. For starters, you can do them with your back rounded, and then flatten the back as you progress with exercises. However, exercises will also require a long warm-up.

Overhead Mobility

Overhead mobility exercises relax the muscles in the back of your arms, your upper back, and your shoulders. Passive stretching exercises will improve your overhead mobility, which will help with upper body exercises like handstands. For this, practice these two exercises:

- **Chin-up dead hang,** which stretches your shoulders with external rotation. A basic dead hang has numerous benefits, from decompressing the spine to stretching arm, back, and core muscles. To do a dead hang, step on a bench and grab a secure overhead bar with both of your hands. Your hands should be shoulder-width apart. Step off the bench and hang onto the bar. Hold a relaxed position for ten seconds and up to a minute, if you can. Return to the bench and repeat up to three times. If your beginner shape doesn't yet tolerate this exercise, you can stay on the bench and stretch by grabbing the bar and lifting your chin up. You can then hang onto the bar with your feet resting on the bench.

- **Hanging cobra**, for which you'll need gymnastic rings. Set the height of the rings to match your chest. Grip the rings with your hands. Sink into the hand position slowly by first falling onto your knees, and then pulling the feet and legs backwards into an extended position. Then, slightly twist, first to the side that feels stiffer, and then to the other side. Hold the position for as long as you can and for as long as it feels good. You can also pull your shoulders up and hold for three to five seconds, and then relax. Give this three to five repetitions, then flip to the other position and repeat. To finish, return to the hanging position with your hands aligned with your shoulders, and head parallel with your hands. Hold for a couple of seconds and then step out of the position. This exercise is also great for those who suffer from lower back pain, as well as anyone who wants to stretch their upper back, hands, chest, and lower abdomen.

Overhead positions in calisthenics, such as with handstands, require a great deal of shoulder mobility. As you already learned, stiff shoulders not only limit your movements, but also increase the risk of injury. Overhead mobility ensures stable positioning of your shoulders when exercising, proper overhead flexion, and the ability to extend your elbows while maintaining the stability of your core and spine. As you can see, all areas and body groups are connected, and one can't function well without the strength and flexibility of the other.

Upper body exercises engage your shoulder blade as well, even when exercises don't directly target shoulders. Because of this, your ability to maintain a strong position largely relies on your shoulder stability and range of motion. You need both shoulder stability and range of motion to avoid slumped body positioning. Here are another three simple exercises you can use to boost your overhead mobility:

- **Shoulder mobilization**. For this exercise, simply circle your shoulder through its entire range of motion. Feel tension and crackling? Then circle away until your scapula rotates smoothly and effortlessly!

- **Active end range**. This time, rotate the shoulder with a fully extended arm, using your full range of motion. This exercise boosts your body alignment when doing handstands.

- **Shoulder extension with a band**. This beginner-friendly exercise is easy and fun, and will feel great if your body suffers the consequences of spending work hours behind the desk. Simply stand on a band and grab the upper part of the band with your hands. Extend the band over your head, with hands aligned with your shoulders. From there, stretch the shoulders upwards as much as you can, then bring them down, and then again up so that the shoulders are in a shrugged position. This exercise also engages your lower abdomen and lower back muscles, gently stretches the muscles of your arms, and if you do it while standing on your toes, also stretches lower body muscles and joints.

Chapter 4:

Safety, Rest, and Recovery

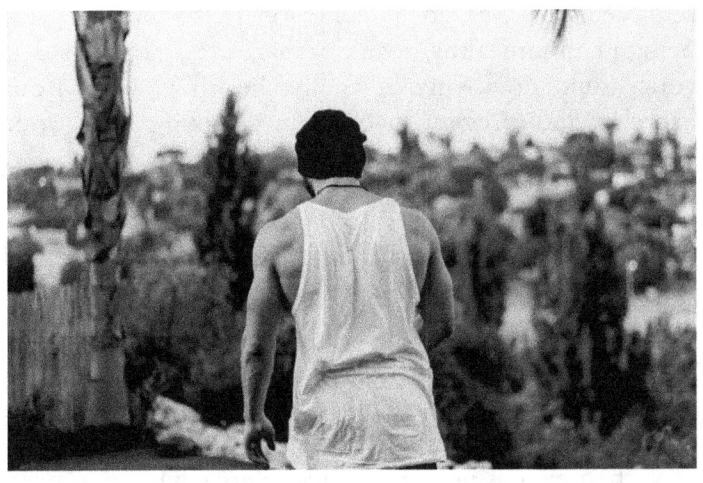

In the previous chapter, you learned about the importance of flexibility and mobility to prevent injuries. However, doing your stretches doesn't guarantee best results and protection from injury. Rest and recovery are also necessary for the greatest health and fitness benefits. In this chapter, you'll learn why rest and recovery lead to better fitness results, and how to rest actively to allow your muscles to grow bigger and stronger.

Safety: How to Prevent Injury in Calisthenics

Injury prevention is an essential part of any training. While calisthenics carries low risk of injury due to the body's limitations in making risky movements and being in an unhealthy position, there are still things that you should do to maximize the health benefits from exercise and prevent overstrain. Training with your bodyweight itself partially prevents overuse, compared to risks with using weights.

Calisthenics training adds less stress to your joints and can lead to fewer injuries, but they can still happen if you're not careful enough. Learning how to prevent injury when exercising calisthenics is necessary if you want to progress consistently. Luckily for you, there are only a couple of simple preventive measures you can use when exercising calisthenics. Here's what you need to do if you want to prevent overstrain when working out:

- **Warm-up**. Never start an exercise session without warming up for at least 10 minutes. Bodyweight training is often thought to be light enough as to not require warm-ups by beginners, and taking extra 10 minutes to do it may seem like taking away from your exercise routine. This isn't true. A proper warm-up will boost your progress and make exercise easier and more enjoyable. I suggested a couple of interesting warm-up exercises for flexibility and mobility in the previous chapter. However, you can still choose any warm-up exercise you like. Warming up is necessary for the blood to start running through your joints and lubricating them to prevent injury.

- **Practice with a lacrosse ball**. Calisthenics doesn't require much equipment or lifting aids, but a couple of useful tools, a lacrosse ball being one of them, will maximize your exercise and performance. A lacrosse ball is useful to protect your joints from injury, particularly those in your elbows and wrists. Massaging these areas with a lacrosse ball helps remove joint pain and ease the stress from these areas. You can easily remove any joint or muscle pain by simply rolling the ball on the spots where you feel soreness, tightness, or tension. If you do this regularly, you will easily prevent post-workout muscle and joint soreness.

- **Use progressions**. Start with lighter variations of more demanding exercises first to allow your muscles and joints enough time to warm up. For example, if you want to do handstands, do a couple of regular push-ups first. Only a couple of repetitions are enough to adapt your body to the movement. This way, you will prevent overstraining joints.

- **Shuffle target areas**. You should switch exercises to target different muscle groups within your workout sessions. Doing so will prevent muscles from adapting to a certain movement, which will reduce its effectiveness. Secondly, you will avoid adding too much tension on your joints, which can happen if you do too many repetitions of the same exercise. For this, it's best to come up with two weekly exercise variations. Plan for two different exercise patterns targeting desired muscle groups, and then rotate these routines. This will also keep you from being bored with your exercises, which can happen if you use the same routine session after session and week after week.

- **Focus on skills**. Calisthenics is different from weight lifting in many ways, one of them being that the progress happens due to improved physical skills, and not cranking up certain exercises and repetitions. Focusing on learning physical movements, rather than on exterior results, shifts your focus from the visual appearance of your body to a sense of inner, instinctive need to improve your body's shape and mobility. This way, when you observe your arm, for example, you won't think only about what you want the biceps and triceps to look like. When you pay attention to adding weight to your exercises and increasing repetitions, you fail to think about how it aligns with your unique physique and health. This can lead to injury.

Instead, focus on the type of movement you're trying to conquer, and ways to learn it. Muscles will grow from this approach most definitely, but focusing on the accuracy of movement, proper position, and alignment of your body will give not only better physical results, but also greater health benefits. It also prevents injuries, because your thinking revolves around the needs and limitations of your body.

Calisthenics Rest and Recovery

If your goal is to build muscle strength, become more flexible and vital, and improve overall shape and health, then resting may sound counterintuitive. It's particularly difficult not to exercise if you're high in energy, you love it, and have started seeing your first results. Still, rest and recovery are vital. They allow your muscles and connective tissues to recover and grow, and also to avoid overload. Here's a simple explanation of why.

When you exercise correctly, and even with the best exercise plan possible, your muscles and connective tissues suffer micro-tears. This minor damage done to the muscles actually produces muscle growth, because the body "fills" these tears to heal the muscle, causing it to grow in size. However, this can't happen, at least not healthily, without rest and recovery. The pattern is simple: add strain and stress to your muscles to create these minor tears, and then rest to let them heal and let your muscles grow.

The philosophy behind rest and recovery is simple, but its execution usually isn't. Beginner calisthenics exercisers are mainly confused about how often and for how long to exercise, and how long to rest and recover afterward. Other questions that puzzle exercisers also concern proper diet during workout and rest days, which we'll address in one of the following chapters.

For the time being, let's focus on the importance of rest and recovery. You may feel great after an intense workout, but your body is, in fact, exhausted and drained. The progression happens after exercising, when your brain and body start to adapt to the new circumstances. When your brain detects intense physical stress, it will trigger adaptation processes during the time you're resting. However, if you don't rest enough, you risk injury. If you overstrain consistently and for long periods of time, you risk injuring yourself so much that you're unable to train for up to a year.

Doing calisthenics will place a huge amount of stress on your body. It adds stress not only to muscles, but also connective tissues, wrists, and ligaments. As you already learned, they take nearly twice as long to recover compared to muscles. Regular calisthenics exercisers frequently suffer from elbow pain and pain in forearms. If this happens, one of the ways to ease the pain is to stop training for a while and rest. This will release the tightness from injured tissues. If you rest regularly after training throughout weeks and months, you'll be able to exercise for years without injury. However, if you suffer a severe injury, it could stop you from exercising overall.

There are many reasons why people refuse to rest. Some feel like missing out on every opportunity to exercise will make them lose strength or put weight back on. Others simply want to take every chance they can to improve, or have become addicted to training because it's satisfying and stimulating. If you're training for a competition, it's possible for a deadline to push you into overtraining.

While all of these reasons are often hard to resist, there are also numerous valid reasons for taking a rest, despite feeling reluctant to do so. First things first, up to a week of rest won't cause you to lose strength. Instead, you could gain even more strength due to adaptation. When you rest, your muscles heal and grow.

However, it's important to adjust your diet to new circumstances to avoid weight gain.

Structured rest can even help you achieve better results. If you rest regularly and consistently between exercises, your neural and muscular systems will better adapt to the new stress. This process is called supercompensation, and it is a physiological response that happens when you get much stronger than you were.

If you become addicted to training, it can become unhealthy and dangerous, both physically and mentally. Taking some time off training will help your body and mind discover and gain a better perspective and balance.

If you're getting ready for a sporting event or a competition, your exercise program needs to include enough rest. If you fail to rest, it will only hurt your performance. Now that you know why you should rest, let's discuss how you should rest and recover from training properly.

How to Plan Calisthenics Rest Days

You should plan your rest days according to your exercise goals and intensity. The more intense and regular the exercise, the more time will be needed to rest and adapt. This means that rest days should be evenly distributed throughout your weekly plan.

What are Rest Days?

As the name suggests, rest days are the days of the week when you won't be training. You should be realistic and flexible when planning your rest days. This is a highly individual matter, and you should take enough time to decide whether you should rest every other or every third day. This will depend on your lifestyle and activity, your recovery ability, your health, and your schedule. However, this plan shouldn't be too strict. You should allow yourself more time to rest if you feel like you need it.

But how do you start making your ideal resting schedule? Typical exercise plans for regular exercisers may not be suitable for calisthenics beginners, so you'll need a lighter pace. If you're just starting, your muscles, ligaments, and tendons will take longer to recover compared to seasoned exercisers. To prevent injury, it might be good to opt-in for longer rest periods between upper body exercises.

Aside from this, you should also plan for so-called de-load weeks. Your plan is best done across four weeks, with week four being lighter and lower in volume compared to the previous three. This, however, doesn't mean that the exercises should be too light, or that you should stop training completely during that week. The intensity of exercises should remain adequate to maintain progress, but with a slightly lower exercise volume and stress. During this week, you can focus more on mobility and flexibility exercises. Rest assured that these lower-stress exercises won't hurt your performance. Chances are that, after you've followed through with the correct plan, you will come back stronger and more flexible.

In this chapter, you learned more about the significance of rest and recovery in calisthenics. During rest days, your body will recover and strengthen itself. Rest is anything but the loss of precious time for exercise. In fact, as you learned, if you exercise continuously without rest, it can actually weaken you and cause long-term muscle damage. You learned that rest days are necessary for both physiological and psychological reasons. It's not only that your muscles need time to rebuild and strengthen, but you also need time to unwind from training, and to balance fitness with home and work. In fact, if you don't rest enough, you can even suffer from overtraining syndrome.

As you learned, recovery is the time when your body adapts to the stress it experienced, and that's the time when muscle strengthening and growth happen. This is also the time for you to recover the water lost from sweat and prevent dehydration, and for your muscles to replenish their glycogen supplies and energy stores, and grow by repairing the damaged tissue. In the short-term, recovery, if active, will replenish your energy for long-term exercise and progress. Long-term, it will help your body adapt to physical exercise and contribute to strengthening your muscles so that you can progress.

Chapter 5:

Rebalance the Scales

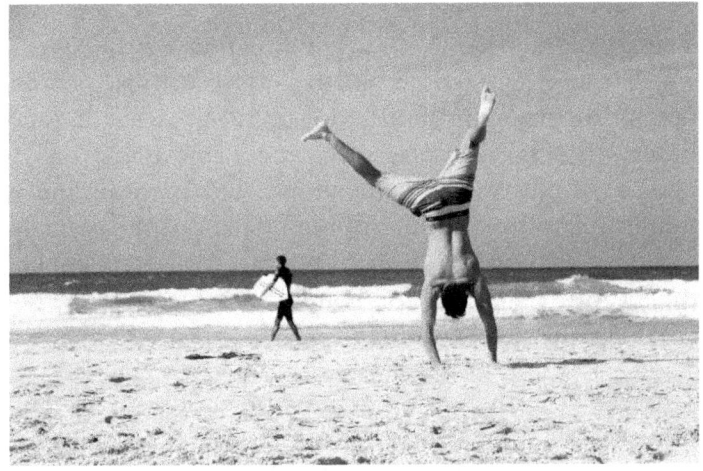

Calisthenics is a form of exercise that combines strength, endurance, mobility, and gymnastic exercise under one umbrella. In the introduction, we discussed why this form of exercise appeals to so many people of different ages, fitness levels, and health levels.

What makes calisthenics so amazing is that it is not just exercising that brings a wide spectrum of different benefits for every practitioner, but it is also a complete lifestyle change. As their bodies change physically, their way of eating changes, and they live a healthier and far more active lifestyle. Their mental health and emotional well-being transform, and they approach everything in their lives with mindfulness.

Life Lessons

The word calisthenics is a combination of the Greek words meaning strength and beauty. For most people, the word strength points to physical strength, and beauty means the pleasing outer appearance of a person. While this is true, these words mean much more than just physical attributes. Think of the strength of determination to go on in the face of adversity, and the beauty of caring for someone without expecting anything in return.

Physical calisthenics teaches practitioners certain fundamental life skills that do not involve physical prowess or physical strength, but have a great impact in other areas of their lives.

Discipline

We live in a world of instant gratification, where we press a button and we get what we want. Everyone multitasks, and often we do not really concentrate on any one thing at a time. Technology has spoiled us, and also robbed us of the vital life skills we all need.

When you start on your journey of calisthenics, you have a goal or goals in mind of what you want to achieve. You know you need physical fitness to achieve whatever goals you have set, but you also need mental discipline to achieve those goals.

It takes discipline to keep going when you are tired, or when you are not succeeding in a specific goal, even though you are trying very hard. Calisthenics helps you to develop discipline through the determination to reach your goals and make the targets you have set for yourself.

As your mindset develops to succeed, so does your mental discipline with each step you take forward. A chain reaction happens when you become determined to succeed. At the end of the day, the determination and discipline you have developed carry over into all other areas of your life. Your education, your career, and your personal life all benefit from strong mental discipline.

Learn to Manage the Fear of Failure

Practicing calisthenics teaches you how to manage the fear of failing at doing something. As you progress in your training, you will face failure when you don't have enough energy to complete the sets and reps you have as your goal. You will fail when you can't smoothly execute a specific hold and you end up falling. This is part of making progress in calisthenics.

Learning to accept that failure does not mean the end, but instead that it is a learning curve, is how you progress in your training and in other areas of your life. Take this lesson from calisthenics and apply it to other areas of your life. You do not have to fear failure. Embrace it, dust yourself off, and try again. You are learning, not failing. Look for and find solutions to achieve your goals.

Self-Control

Calisthenics training teaches you how to control your body physically. You'll learn how to lift it, push, and maneuver it in many different ways that you could not do before. The philosophy of self-mastery that calisthenics is based on is not a new concept. Many of the ancient religious philosophies of the world are based upon this. Self-mastery through calisthenics training extends past just the physical, to achieve mastery over our emotions and desires. Learning and achieving self-control of your emotions and desires benefits your entire life. It affects how you handle situations, and how you respond to not only good, but also bad stimuli.

Self-Reliance

People have different ways in which they strive to maintain fitness and health. They go to the gym and use the rowing machine and the treadmill, or they lift weights or use cross training equipment. They benefit greatly from this, and there is nothing wrong with their chosen methods. Yet, using these machines and equipment means they rely on external tools to maintain their levels of fitness. Remove their equipment, and suddenly everything comes to a halt.

With calisthenics, you only rely on yourself. You are not lost without a trainer or a treadmill. You only need your own body to achieve your fitness goals. You learn self-reliance without dependence on any externals.

This applies to your life in general. Think about how often you have heard someone say that they cannot feel good unless they can buy expensive things. Maybe a friend has remarked to you that they cannot feel good about themselves unless they have their partner's or their boss' approval. They have not learned to be self-reliant.

Calisthenics teaches you that you only have to rely on yourself to achieve fitness and good health, and that you already have yourself to make you feel good. All you need to do is learn how to correctly use your body and your mind.

Physical Benefits

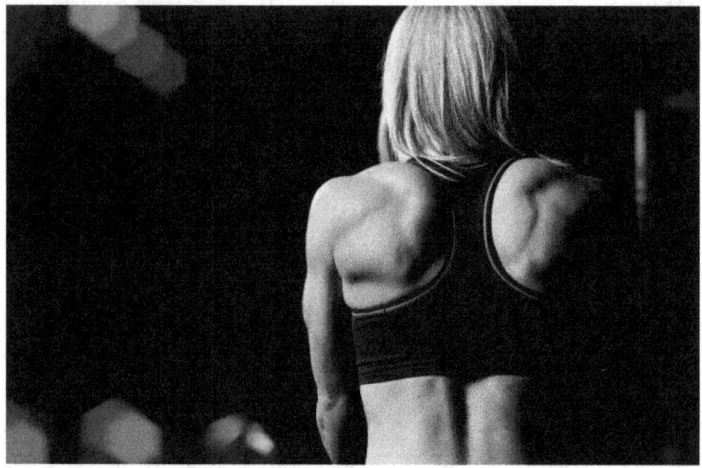

Doing consistent calisthenics workouts has far-reaching health benefits for any practitioner. The health benefits are short-term and long-term, as many of the benefits become very important over time. Calisthenics practitioners experience a much better quality of life as they grow older.

The following benefits definitely make calisthenics worthwhile, even if it seems to be difficult at times:

Bone Density

Calisthenics promotes an increase in bone density, which is crucially important to prevent or reduce the risk of developing osteoporosis.

Chronic Conditions

Consistent calisthenics workouts help to control or prevent several chronic conditions that could be life-threatening, such as:

- Obesity
- Diabetes
- Arthritis
- Back pain
- Heart disease
- Depression
- High blood pressure
- High cholesterol
- Osteoporosis
- Certain forms of cancer

- Stroke

Cognitive Decline

Physical and mental discipline through exercise may prevent or reduce the effects of cognitive decline in senior citizens.

Energy Levels

As you progress with calisthenics, you'll grow stronger, and your energy levels will increase quite noticeably.

Flexibility, Mobility, and Balance

Calisthenics helps you to maintain balance and flexibility through increased mobility. This is important as your body ages in order to stay independent and agile.

Greater Stamina

Calisthenics creates a chain reaction of increased physical activity, strength building, better health, and wellbeing that all contribute to increased stamina.

Immune System

High levels of fitness and a nutritionally balanced diet assists the immune system to fight off illnesses.

Insomnia and Sleep

Increased fitness levels and improved mental wellbeing promotes better sleep patterns and greatly reduces the problem of insomnia.

Muscle Strength and Tone

Increased protection of your joints from injury comes with enhanced muscle strength.

Performance of Everyday Tasks

With calisthenics, you build functional strength, and not just strength for lifting heavy weights or putting muscles on display. Lean, functional muscles make doing everyday tasks much easier, with less strain on muscles and joints.

Posture

Increased muscle strength and flexibility improves posture greatly.

Risk of Injury

The risk of injury decreases with progression, muscle building, and increased strength.

Self-Esteem

When you follow a consistent workout program and you can see the improvements you are making through mastering your physical body, it increases your self-esteem.

Sense of Wellbeing

Resistance training may have a boosting effect on self-confidence and developing a positive body image. An increase in your sense of wellbeing promotes a positive mood.

Weight-Management and Muscle to Fat Ratio

Consistent workouts increase your muscle mass and burn calories even while you are at rest. This makes weight management much easier.

Mental and Emotional Wellbeing

Every human wants to be happy. In fact, happiness is part of human DNA, through a protein created by the FAAH gene that affects pain and pleasure. The best way to show you how calisthenics contributes to your mental and emotional wellbeing is to share the Action for Happiness movement's GREAT DREAM, or the 10 keys to happier living. Calisthenics ties directly in with each of the 10 keys, with great potential to improve your life and wellbeing.

Giving

Calisthenics gives you the opportunity to give to others by sharing your skills and experiences as you progress. You give your time, a precious commodity, to help others by sharing what you have learned on your own journey and to encourage others to start calisthenics training.

Relating

The calisthenics community is very close-knit in comparison with other health and fitness groups. Calisthenics is mostly non-competitive and has a culture of sharing and openness that promotes camaraderie. This is helpful especially for beginners to connect with others who share their passion, and find a lot of moral support is freely offered.

Exercising

Our bodies are not designed to live a sedentary life. Our bodies are designed for movement. The more movement we engage in, the more our bodies release endorphins, or the happiness hormone in layman's terms. So yes, when you exercise your body thanks you by releasing endorphins that make you feel good and give you an all-around sense of wellbeing.

Appreciating

Calisthenics offers practitioners two different ways in which they experience appreciation. The first way is that you literally are able to get outside to do your workouts. You are not bound to work out in a specific building or a specific environment. Depending on where you live, you may have nature at your doorstep, or you could enjoy doing your sets and reps in a beautiful park. Wherever you live, you can breathe in the fresh air while you enjoy the world around you at the same time.

The second way is through mindfulness. Calisthenics, as we said before, is not only physical exercises. It involves your mind, sharpens your focus, and hones your mental discipline. When you focus on your workout and striving toward your next goal, you do not waste brainpower worrying and stressing about things in your life that irk you, or that you can't really do anything about.

Trying Out

Doing calisthenics means that you never stop learning. There is always the next goal, or honing a specific skill. The potential for learning new things is literally endless, as you can keep on exploring new movements every time you have mastered one.

Direction

Every person needs goals to look forward to in their life, or something to strive for. This is part of human nature, and we are at our happiest when we have clearly defined goals of where we want to go. Calisthenics offers many goals you can achieve through determination, diligence, and effort.

Resilience

In the section titled Life Lessons, we discussed the management of the fear of failure. This is the mental health skill calisthenics teaches you, resilience and finding ways to bounce back again when you have failed. The physical hardships and failures you experience through training help to develop resilience to deal with failures in other aspects of your life. As your body develops, you'll learn about yourself and the ability you have to overcome whatever obstacles are in your way. This carries over to your personal relationships, your career, family, and friends.

How to Balance Healthy Eating Socially

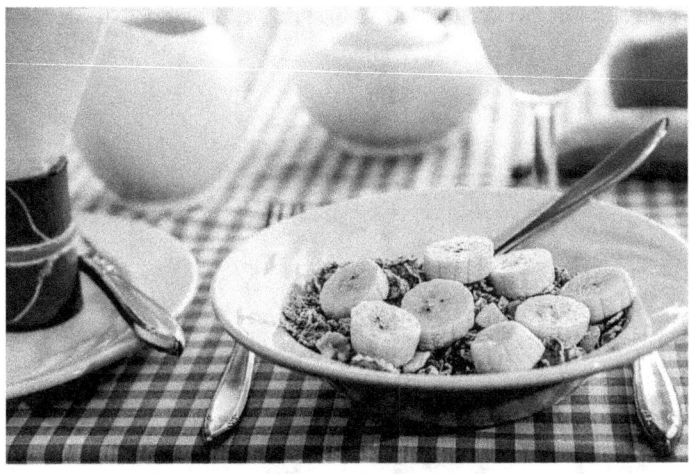

Socializing and eating out can be harrowing for anyone still at the beginning of their calisthenics training. You work very hard for every step forward, and eating out with friends and colleagues can wipe out many hours of hard work. This sets you back and can drain your motivation, and nobody needs that. That is why it is good to have a handful of tips to help avoid the pitfalls for socializing and eating out when you are committed to building a healthy body and mind through calisthenics.

Check the Menu

Check out what is available on the menu before the meeting time. This avoids having to choose food when you might be very hungry or tired, and making unhealthy food choices on the spur of the moment.

Healthy Snack Before Arrival

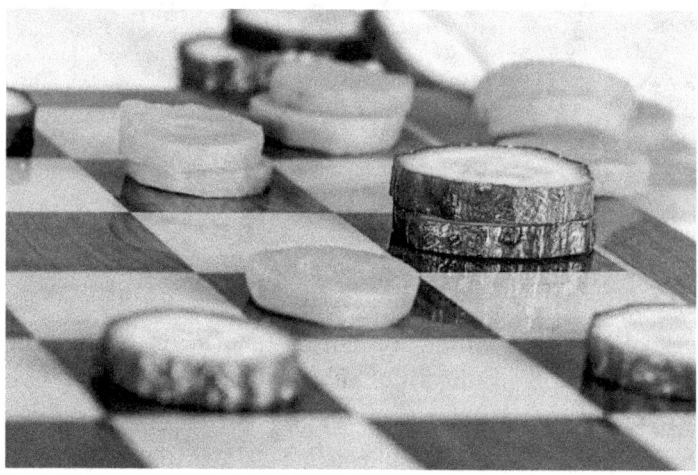

When we are very hungry, we tend to overeat. If we eat out at a place where the wait for food to be served may be long, this could lead to wrong food choices and eating too much. Eat a high protein, healthy snack such as yogurt or a smoothie before you go to the restaurant.

Water

Keep a glass of water handy at all times. Drink water before the start of the meal and during, and have water instead of a sweetened drink. You will save yourself from a lot of extra calories.

Check How Food is Prepped and Cooked

The way food is prepared and cooked can have a huge impact on the number of calories and fat content of a dish. Buzz words to look for are sautéed, crispy, pan-fried, crunchy, and fried, as these dishes are usually higher in fat content and calories. Rather, look for steamed, poached, grilled, and roasted items on the menu.

Order First

We are often influenced by what other people at the table order when eating out in a group. The best way to avoid temptation and any uncomfortable moments is simply to order your food before anyone else can.

Double Up on Appetizers

Some restaurants specialize in serving huge portions, and that could mean overeating. The best way to avoid this problem is to order two appetizers instead of a huge main course. You will eat enough to be full, without an overload of calories.

Mindful Eating

Mindful eating changes eating habits, and is very helpful in social settings where overeating and bad food choices are abundant. Mindful eating means you savor each flavor and aroma of each mouthful of food, and concentrate on what feelings you experience as you taste each different piece of food. According to findings in a 2013 study, mindful eating helps gain self-control that prevents overeating, and aids in making healthier food choices when eating at social events and restaurants (Robinson et al.).

Eat Slowly and Chew Well

This tip to cope with eating out works hand-in-hand with mindful eating. By consciously slowing down how fast you eat and trying to chew each mouthful of food X number of times, your body has ample time to signal fullness before you overeat.

Coffee Instead of Dessert

Bypass the dessert trap and order a cup of coffee instead. This will greatly cut your calorie count, and you will actually enjoy the surprisingly many health benefits that coffee has.

Request a Healthy Swap

When you place your order, request to swap out high-calorie items such as potatoes, fries, and pan-fried or sautéed items. Replace these items with vegetables or a salad.

Dressings and Sauces on the Side

Make it a habit to always ask that any sauces and dressings for the food you order be served on the side. Sauces and dressings are notoriously high in fats and calories, and you can control how much you have much more easily when it is served on the side.

Bread Basket

The bread basket offered before dinner is standard practice at many restaurants. If you are already hungry when you arrive, you will be very tempted to nibble and throw your eating plan out the door. Rather, send the bread basket back and avoid temptation.

Salad or Soup Starters

A 2007 study has shown that you can lower your overall calorie intake at a meal by as much as 20% when you start with soup (Flood & Rolls, 2007). The findings also showed that this works no matter what type of soup you have. This is a great way to save on calories and give you peace of mind about not interrupting your training program.

Share or Go Half-Portion

People who practice portion control often share food with another person at the table. It is a convenient way to prevent overeating, and it helps both people. If there is nobody to share with, ask the waiter for a half-portion of your order. Most restaurants will allow you to order half-portions. If they don't then, tell them to pack up half your food for you to take home in a doggy bag.

Alcohol, Mixers, and Sweetened Drinks

Nobody said you have to avoid all forms of alcohol when you socialize. You simply have to think ahead and do things logically. Order a small glass of wine instead of a large glass, and ask for a diet mixer when your spirits instead of a mixer sweetened with sugar.

Soft drinks can also push up calories when eating out. It is much healthier to drink water, natural unsweetened drinks, or a cup of unsweetened tea.

Tomato-Based vs. Creamy Sauces

Try to steer clear of cheese sauces, and any sauces made with cream. Rather, go for the much healthier option of tomato-based or vegetable-based sauces for a great-tasting and much lower calorie sauce.

Be Wary of Health Claims

It is not uncommon these days to see items listed on restaurant menus as "sugar-free", "keto", "gluten-free", or "paleo". Always keep in mind that sugar-free only means there is no cane sugar in the product or dish, and most of the time other forms of sweeteners have been used that are the same or higher in calories than sugar.

It is the same with items highlighted as fulfilling the needs of certain diets, as some diets are incredibly high in fats. So, have a good read through the menu and never fall for the hype.

Chapter 6:

The Fuel for Lean Living

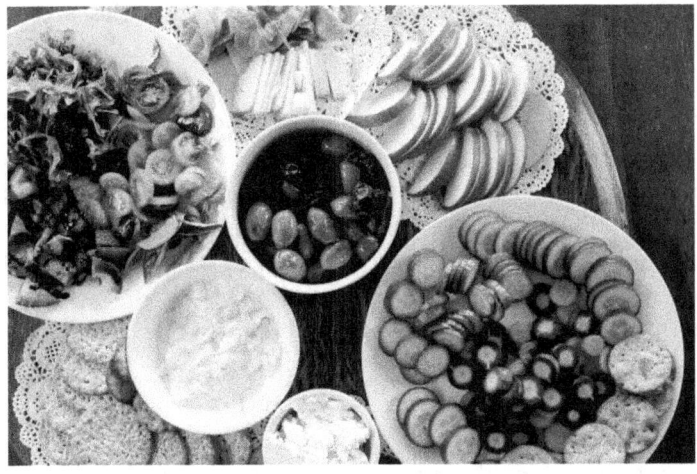

Building your body up will require a suitable diet. Well, health and wellbeing in general require a healthy diet to begin with. It's important to remember that the way you eat affects your capacity to exercise and the result of it, from before you start your exercise plan, during exercise, and while you're resting.

How much you'll have to adjust your diet depends on how proper your diet is now. If you come from a place of over or undereating and you can't maintain a regular, healthy eating schedule, your first step will be to establish a proper diet plan. Unless you eat well, you won't have enough energy to exercise, or you will, but the results will fail to show.

From the standpoint of achieving hypertrophy, or gaining muscle, your diet will have to keep up with your schedule. On the other hand, your diet mustn't be too rigorous either. You'll face life outside dieting and exercising, and daily activities and life hurdles won't care much for your need to eat properly. You'll need a simple, well-composed, sustainable, and practical diet if you want it to work for you long-term. A rigorous diet will be hard to keep up with, regardless of its perceived health and fitness benefits. Adopting a healthy diet is best done step-by-step, one day at a time, the same way as starting to exercise. We want you to be successful with your transformation, and we know that people can't tolerate too many sudden changes.

Can you slip into a strict diet and exercise schedule that's completely different than you used to have? Likely not. Health and fitness are gained one step at a time, even if it means that, on your first day, you'll exercise for only ten minutes and give up candy. Those are the kinds of little changes that snowball into a complete life transformation. One day, it's doing ten squats and switching regular pizza with the lean substitute. The next day, it will be ten lunges and two pushups, and you may eat a smoothie for breakfast instead of your usual sugary cereal. Fast forward a year from now, and you're a different person. So, be patient with yourself and snowball into your transformation.

For starters, adjusting to a healthy diet for calisthenics means introducing regular, healthy changes in your meal sizes, food choices, and eating schedule. But first, you need to think about your body, health, lifestyle, and goals to decide what kind of diet you need. Start by calculating how many calories you need on your exercise days and your resting days. Next, consider your training goal when developing a meal plan, either:

- **Muscle gain**. If you've chosen calisthenics to gain muscles, your daily calorie intake will have to be bigger than the number of calories you spend. On average, you should add 200-500 calories to your daily diet.

- **Fat loss**. If your goal is to lose fat, you should make a calorie deficit of between 200 and 500 calories in your daily diet. However, you still need to make sure that your food intake is sufficient to support daily physical activity. Remember, you'll be physically active even on your rest days, and eating too little might slow down your metabolism.

General Diet Recommendations

Eating a healthy diet for successful calisthenics shouldn't be difficult. This section will give you a couple of simple dietary recommendations to follow.

- **Focus on food quality.** Postulates of a healthy diet are often vague, and they entail eating an abundance of lean meats, healthy carbs, and vegetables. However, you also need to make sure to have enough food to keep you running. Don't fall into a trap of reducing protein, carbs, and fat to below limits just because you want to get slimmer. You still need your meats, rice, and oats, even if you're trying to lose weight. On the other hand, your diet needs to be versatile and satisfying as well. You won't feel good if you only eat lean, cooked foods, with complete disregard for your personal tastes. You can allow yourself to eat cheat meals and have some of the delicious foods you otherwise enjoy, because this will provide a break from being on a strict regimen and help you feel like all of the effort is worth it.

- **Pay attention to your appetite.** Designing your meals according to calorie charts may distract you from paying attention to your real appetite. It is possible to have a strong appetite and eat a lot but be unable to gain weight, and to have a low appetite and eat little, but still be unable to lose weight. Neither of the possibilities are excluded. If it happens that you eat a lot without weight gain, pay attention to whether or not you're eating enough protein, and also if you're overtraining. It's possible that you need more rest for hypertrophy. On the other hand, if you reduce your diet, but you're still not losing weight, it's possible that you're eating too little. In that case, you might feel sluggish and exhausted, and not even feel the appetite under the influence of overstrain. Again, revisit your diet and exercise plan to see if calorie intake and diet composition match your daily calorie expenditure. It can also happen that you don't have enough appetite for your target calorie intake. If you struggle with appetite, you can choose more calorie-dense foods to consume a greater number of nutrients with smaller food quantities. On top of that, you can also reduce fiber intake, because fibers from oats and rice are known to reduce appetite.

- **Be careful with protein supplements.** Eating a diet that's well-aligned with your exercise should supply enough protein for muscle growth and strengthening. You should only consider protein supplements if you have certain dietary restrictions, or you otherwise struggle with eating meat, eggs, and dairy.

Diet Plan Ideas

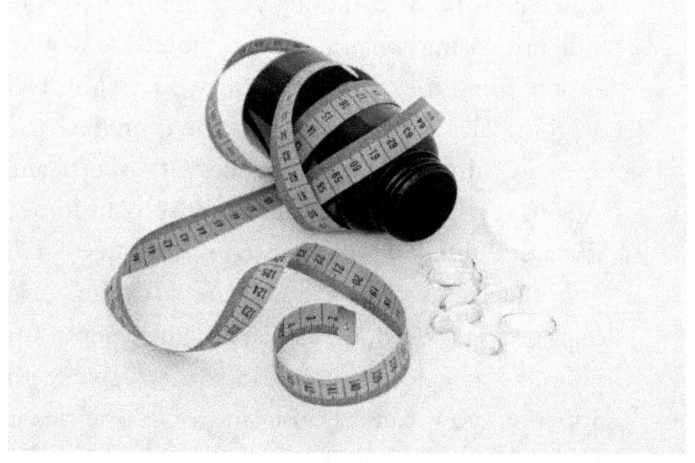

Quality nutrition is necessary for optimal fitness results, with calisthenics as well as with any other training program. Not having a good nutrient balance will get in the way of your fitness goals, regardless of your effort. If you're not used to following a specific diet program, understanding how you need to eat for healthy results with calisthenics could be a challenge. For that reason, this section will provide a diet plan that's best to follow when you're exercising calisthenics. This plan won't specify exactly what you need to eat or give precise food quantities. Instead, it will give you general guidelines for a healthy diet that supports regular exercise. With this plan, it will be easy to adjust food choices and portion sizes according to your daily needs.

To follow a diet suitable for calisthenics exercise, there's no need for you to invest in cooking equipment or fancy foods. There's also no need to spend more on food than you used to, or adjust your schedule to have enough time to cook. This diet plan will be flexible and allow you to adjust it to your individual taste and preference, as well as to your fitness goals. Weighing your food is one of the easier ways to adjust meal sizes and avoid under or overeating. Here are the basic directions to eat healthily when practicing calisthenics.

- **Eat whole foods**. You'll get the best nutrition with unprocessed foods. Processed foods don't only contain toxic chemicals. They are also heavily processed to have a longer shelf life, so they're depleted of precious nutrients that you need in order to grow your muscles and strength. Instead, get your macronutrients from organic meat, fish, dairy, seafood, and eggs. Fruits and vegetables will provide natural fibers and carbs from sugar, and grains and root vegetables will supply healthy carbs as well.

- **Cut out unhealthy food**. You need to stop eating junk food and processed fats if you want to be healthy in general, but also if you want to make progress with calisthenics. In addition to that, you should also eliminate white rice and all products made from white flour, including pastries and pasta.

- **Don't limit fruits and vegetables**. You can have as many plants as you want, and it won't get in the way of your health or exercise results.

- **Limit mealtimes**. You shouldn't scatter your meals across the entire day. Instead, eat within an eight-hour feeding window. This will help you eat when you're hungry without restrictions, but still prevent you from getting too hungry. If you don't go hungry, there's less chance that you'll feel tempted to eat junk foods. Instead, you'll eat foods that are more calorie-dense, and consume fewer calories than if you spread your meals across the entire day.

- **Supplement cautiously**. You should aim to get the majority of your nutrition from your daily meals, not supplements. In case you still feel like you'd benefit from supplementation, you should use the following supplements cautiously:

- **Creatine**. Creatine will help you recover from injuries and supports building muscle mass.

- **Proteins**. If you feel like you can't eat sufficient protein to build muscles, or you're a vegetarian or a vegan, then supplemental protein will be a great substitute for meat. It will also help injured muscles recover in case you over train.

- **Branched-chain amino acids**, or BCAA, can help you gain muscle and maintain the muscle growth you achieved so far.

- **Vitamins**. Although you will easily eat sufficient vitamins when consuming fruits and vegetables, multivitamin supplementation can help obtain those nutrients that are otherwise hard to gain through diet, like Zinc, B complex, and vitamins E, D, and C.

To understand how to eat healthily when doing calisthenics, you should first learn how to balance out macronutrients in your diet. Your carbs, fats, and protein require a good proportion in your meals for optimal performance effects. Here's how to eat to get sufficient healthy macronutrients:

- **Carbohydrates.** You should focus on eating complex carbohydrates, which won't spike your blood sugar and cause excess blood glucose to be stored in fat cells. You'll find complex carbs in fruits and vegetables, whole grains, and nuts and seeds. Fiber from fruits and vegetables also breaks down into carbohydrates when consumed.

- **Fats.** Aside from fats naturally found in meat, dairy, nuts, and seeds, you should also use healthy fats while cooking. Ideal choices include extra virgin olive oil and coconut oil. Saturated fats are found in meats and tropical plants like coconuts, while unsaturated fats are present in fish, nuts, and vegetables. You should reduce your intake of saturated fats by choosing lean meats, because human bodies can produce them on their own. However, essential fatty acids, like omega 3 and omega 6, must be obtained through diet. This is why it's advised to have at least two servings of fish each week, and to use scarce amounts of extra virgin olive oil when cooking. Still, even these fats can cause obesity when consumed in excess amounts.

- **Proteins.** Proteins form your muscles, nails, hair, and ligaments, and serve to keep your body moving. They are amino acids that serve as building blocks for muscles. When looking for sources of healthy protein, look for lean meats and fish, but also lean dairy, eggs, mushrooms, legumes, and beans. These foods can be eaten in large amounts without contributing to weight gain.

- **Micronutrients.** Last but not least are vitamins and minerals found in fruits and vegetables. Vitamins are necessary to support biological processes in your body, and in terms of calisthenics, they secure strong and safe movements. Vitamin deficiency often affects metabolism, your energy levels, and your appearance.

Eating Tips and Meal Ideas

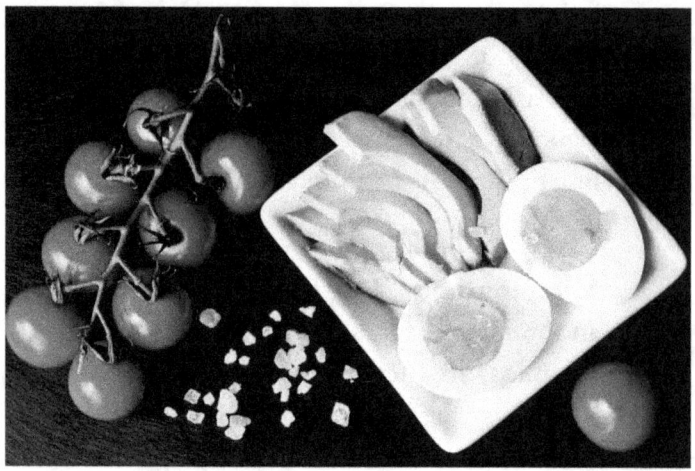

So far, we've given you general recommendations for how to eat properly when practicing calisthenics. In this section, you'll find a couple of meal ideas for breakfast to dinner, to help you get a sense of what your daily meals should look like.

Breakfast

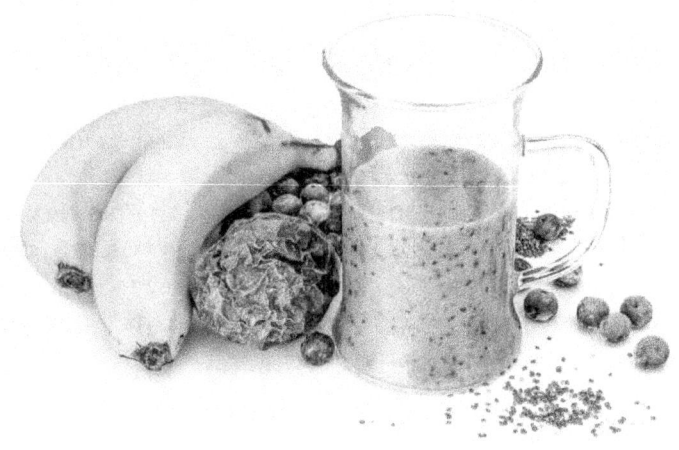

Oatmeal with Fruit

Ingredients:

- 1-2 cups whole oats
- 1-2 cups regular, almond, or coconut milk
- 1 cup berries
- Up to 1 cup crushed nuts

Instructions:

You need a strong breakfast to get you going, and oatmeal with berries of your choice (strawberries, blueberries, or mixed berries,) with the addition of fruits like bananas, mangoes, and oranges, is a great option. One bowl is usually a good measure regardless of gender and lifestyle, but you can adjust your breakfast to add or reduce calories as needed. For example, if you want a leaner breakfast, go for coconut or almond milk instead of regular, or cut back on the fruit serving. On the other hand, if you want to increase the caloric value of the dish, you can add up to a cup of nuts. Keep in mind that nuts are calorie-dense and could add up to 200 calories to a meal. Berries and fruits are important to supply enough sugar, but in a healthy way, and of course to add fiber that supports the health of your digestive system.

Fruit Salad

Ingredients:

- Chopped fruits (bananas, avocado, apples, oranges, pineapple, strawberries, or raspberries)
- 1 tbsp. raw honey
- 1 tbsp. lemon juice

Instructions:

If you prefer a lighter breakfast, you can have as many bananas, avocados, oranges, berries, apples, and citruses as you please. The secret to eating the right amount of fruit is simple: chew and eat slowly, and only eat to the point where you feel full.

Breakfast Tortilla

Ingredients:

- 1 whole wheat tortilla

For fruit topping:

- 1 cup chopped fruit
- 1 tbsp. peanut or almond butter
- Up to 1 cup crushed nuts

For vegetable topping:

- Chopped vegetables (tomatoes, spinach, kale, or onions)
- A drizzle of olive oil
- 1 tbsp. lemon juice
- A pinch of salt
- A pinch of pepper
- A pinch of each of the spices of your choosing (parsley, basil, dill, etc.)
- 1 slice cheddar cheese
- Greek yogurt

Instructions:

A whole wheat tortilla is a great breakfast option, regardless of your gender and fitness goals. Your breakfast will be light if you top your tortilla with fruits (berries, bananas, and avocados) or vegetables (sliced tomatoes, leafy greens, olives, cucumber, etc.). If you want to increase the caloric value of your breakfast, you can add a layer of almond or peanut butter if you choose fruits, or add a cup of Greek yogurt to your vegetable wrap. This will add fat to the meal in case you're doing higher volume training. Optionally, you can substitute some of the ingredients with cheddar cheese and kale, or add them if you want to boost your breakfast with extra healthy calories.

Green smoothie

Ingredients:

- 1 handful spinach
- One apple
- 1 handful kale leaves
- One banana
- 1 tbsp. lemon juice
- 1 cup almond or coconut milk
- Water, as needed

Instructions:

Opinions are divided regarding whether or not a smoothie is the best breakfast option. It can be if you add enough carbs to the mix. You can pop any leafy veggies you like into a blender, but an apple with a handful of spinach leaves, some lemon, kale, and a banana is a safe bet. If your smoothie is still too lean, you can add fruit, like a half or a whole banana, or berries to add flavor, vitamins, and calories. Lack of carbs? Add up to a cup of whole oats, and if you're doing high volume training, you can also add a cup of almond or coconut milk. As you can see, there are many healthy ways to add or deduce the caloric volume of your smoothie, and the choice is all yours!

Lunch and Dinner

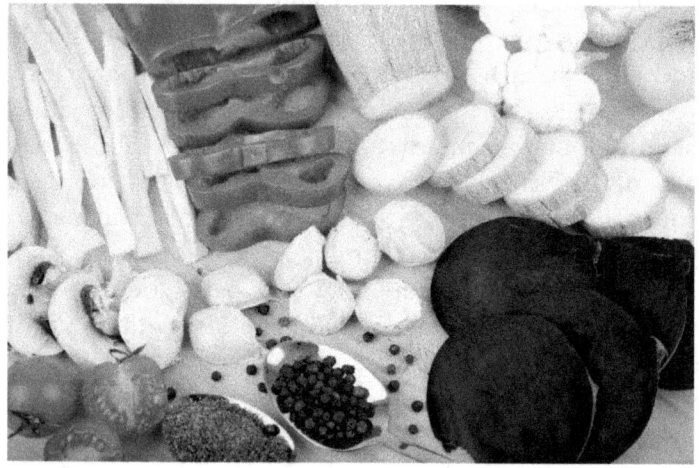

The beauty of healthy cooking is in its versatility. Lunch and dinner combine meats, vegetables, herbs, and spices that can be eaten both during the day and in the evening. For the sake of simplicity, we recommend cooking a double measure of a meal and simply having one serving for lunch, and another for dinner. On the other hand, if you don't want to eat the same meal twice a day, you can always pre-make a couple of meals in advance. Mid-day meals do require a careful balance of carbs and protein. This is because the foods that carry most macronutrients also have quite a bit of fat, and all of that combined can easily spike your blood sugar and make the meal too heavy.

As always, make sure to use whole, organic, non-processed foods. Here are a couple of ideas for healthy, balanced, and satiating meals:

Fish with Vegetables

Ingredients:

- 1 -2 salmon, or any other fish of your choosing (a palm-sized serving)
- 2 cups or more chopped kale, cauliflower, broccoli, onions, zucchini, and eggplant
- 1 tbsp. extra virgin olive oil
- 1 tbsp. lemon juice
- ½ tbsp. chopped parsley
- 1 tsp dill
- 1 tsp basil
- A pinch of salt
- A pinch of pepper

Instructions:

Cooking fish is never too much trouble. If you don't enjoy cooking too much, you can simply grill a palm-sized piece of fish, or boil it. If you want to add flavor, on the other hand, simply top the fish with extra virgin olive oil and sprinkle with spices, like powdered onion, parsley, or dill. For this recipe, you'll make a piece of salmon with a vegetable side-dish made from chopped and sautéed broccoli, spinach, zucchini, cauliflower, and eggplant. Don't forget your avocado! You can have it with your vegetables if you enjoy such a blend, or have it as a dessert.

Meat with Vegetables

Ingredients:

- 1-2 chicken breasts
- 2 or more cups chopped kale, broccoli, spinach, cauliflower, paprika, and zucchini
- Extra virgin olive oil
- A pinch of salt
- A pinch of pepper
- 1 cup vegetable stock
- ½ tbsp. chopped parsley
- ½ tsp basil
- ½ tsp dill
- ½ tsp ginger

Instructions:

The same process for making a healthy, protein-dense meal can be used to cook meat. All you need is a palm-sized piece of meat, which you can grill or chop and sauté however you please! Remember to only use up to one tablespoon of extra virgin olive oil.

To make a side-dish, you can either stir-fry chopped sweet potatoes (up to two cups), or chop veggies of your choosing all together (e.g. kale, broccoli, cauliflower, and spinach), and stir-fry with a little bit of water or a cup of vegetable stock.

Want to spice it up? Add chopped parsley, onions, basil, or dill, or drizzle with a tablespoon of lemon or lime juice.

Beans/Legumes with Stir Fry Vegetables

Ingredients:

- 2 cups quinoa, brown rice, or beans
- 2 cups or more chopped vegetables of your choosing
- One sliced onion
- 1 tbsp. extra virgin olive oil
- A pinch of salt
- A pinch of pepper
- 1 cup vegetable or chicken stock

Instructions:

Now, hold on. Who says you have to eat meat each day to become ripped? Really no one, not even nutritionists. For this meal option, you'll substitute a palm-sized piece of meat with up to two cups of beans or quinoa. Lean meals usually feature a cup-sized measure, while those who want to gain weight and muscle often go for two cups or two small cans.

First, boil your legumes for 30 minutes. They'll be ready to eat, but not very tasty. Grab a pot and add a tablespoon of extra virgin olive oil. Add chopped onions and let simmer briefly, adding a half-a-cup of water or vegetable stock. To increase lean calories, you can use chicken stock. Then, add your rice or quinoa, mix it in, and let simmer for about five minutes. Your meal is nearly finished, and all you need to do is to add up to two cups of finely chopped vegetables, top with more water or stock (up to a glass), and let simmer up to ten more minutes. Enjoy!

In this chapter, you learned how to cook your basic meals to support fitness and muscle growth. But what about your pre-and post-workout snacks? In the next chapter, you'll learn more about the health benefits of smoothies, and how to make them quickly and easily.

Chapter 7:

Getting Started with Smoothies

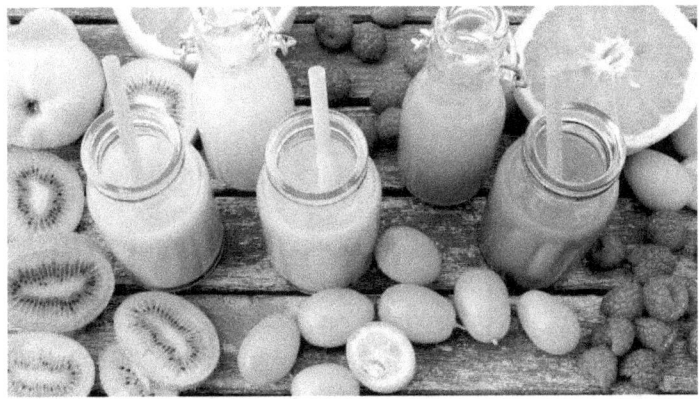

Smoothies are not only for bodybuilders, weight lifters, and dedicated gym junkies. Smoothies are great tasting and pack a protein punch when you need it, whether they are for breakfast, post-workout, or as a delicious snack. The variety you can make is truly endless, and you can adapt the level of sweetness or add savory ingredients as per your personal preference.

A word on protein powders is to take note that protein powder supplements are not FDA regulated. Therefore, the very large number of options and brands available on the market can vary radically from each other. Do your research to find which of the protein powders suits your needs the best.

There are many ways to gear up for making smoothies that will save you time and needless effort. For the majority of people, life is busy, and any possible way to spend less time preparing food is a huge bonus.

Frozen Fruit vs. Fresh

Unless you have a constant supply of fresh fruits and products available at all times, your first shortcut is to start building your supplies of frozen fruits. You can buy containers of frozen fruit in most supermarkets, or you can start your own supply. It is a good idea to freeze your favorite fruits in single-servings in jars, plastic containers, or ziplock bags in the freezer. This way, you can just grab a container and make a smoothie without first having to think about portion sizes.

Make-Ahead Smoothie Packs

You can take your containers of frozen fruit a step further and actually prep your smoothies ahead of time. This is hugely helpful in any household with more than one person using smoothies, as well as an economical step when buying fruit and vegetables in bulk.

Wash and clean all the fruits and vegetables. Then, measure out all the ingredients for each specific smoothie you want to make, and place the ingredients in single smoothie packs in the freezer. The smoothie packs can also be placed in the refrigerator for use within the next few days.

This is the fastest way possible to make a smoothie, as you simply have to add the liquid because all the fruits and veggies have been prepped.

Quick Fix Remedies

Often, we have a smoothie that is either too sweet, too thick, or lacks the amount of tartness you prefer. Here are a couple of quick fixes to help when things go wrong. Add the ingredients to adjust taste or thickness, and blend for an extra 10-20 seconds to incorporate everything.

Too thick: Add a small amount of juice, milk, or water, and blend. Repeat if the mixture is still too thick.

Too thin: Add any of these ingredients to help thicken the mixture:

- Banana
- Strawberries

- Frozen yogurt
- Extra ice
- Chia seeds
- Raw oats
- Protein powder
- Xanthan gum
- Avocado
- Silken tofu
- Nut butter

Bitter taste: Mature greens often have a bitter taste, and the best way to lessen the bitterness is to use baby greens, as they have a much milder taste. You can add any of the following ingredients to lessen the bitterness:

- Bananas, because they have a neutralizing effect on the bitter taste
- Strawberries sweeten green smoothies very well
- Vanilla extract or vanilla bean
- Agave
- Cocoa, or unsweetened cocoa powder

Too sweet: Add frozen lemonade concentrate or fresh lemon juice

Not sweet enough: Add sweeteners or ingredients to sweeten the smoothie little bits at a time, so as to not make it overly sweet. Ingredients include:

- Watermelon, instead of water
- Agave, honey, sugar, or maple syrup
- Stevia, or artificial sweetener of your own choice
- Grapes
- Dates

Not creamy enough: Try any of the ingredients on this list to help create a creamier taste:

- Avocado
- Ice cream
- Vanilla yogurt
- Frozen yogurt

Substitutions

Most smoothie recipes available tell you to use only specific organic ingredients. You can, however, substitute just about any ingredient listed in a smoothie recipe with an ingredient better suitable for your personal needs and tastes. Also, using plant-based ingredients instead makes the recipes vegan and vegetarian friendly.

The following ingredients and their substitutions can be used to mix up really good-tasting protein smoothies that will please everyone.

- Dairy milk
- Soy milk
- Hemp milk
- Almond milk
- Oat milk
- Cashew milk
- Rice milk
- Sorghum milk
- Coconut milk
- Flax milk

- Nuts
- Sunflower seeds, or the butter made from sunflower seeds (sun butter)
- Pumpkin seeds (pepitas)
- Tahini
- Flax seeds
- Chia seeds
- Hemp seeds
- Sugar honey
- Maple syrup
- Brown rice syrup
- Agave nectar
- Barley malt syrup
- Sorghum syrup
- Stevia, or artificial sweetener of your own choice
- Dates
- Grapes

- Whole eggs
- Store-bought Ener-G egg replacement
- 1 tbsp. agar flakes
- 1 tbsp. applesauce
- 1 mashed banana
- ¼ cup silken tofu
- ¼ cup of coconut yogurt
- 1 tbsp. ground flax or chia seeds, simmered for 2 minutes in 3 tbsp. of water (or left to chill in the fridge for 15 minutes)
- Egg whites/aquafaba
- Any of the substitutes listed for whole eggs
- Spinach, bok choy
- Kale
- Radish greens
- Parsley
- Dandelion greens
- Arugula

- Turnip greens
- Celery
- Celery greens
- Collard greens
- Swiss chard
- Mustard greens
- Romaine lettuce
- Broccoli
- Beet greens
- Broccoli rabe (rapini)
- Carrot greens
- Dairy yogurt
- Protein powder
- Coconut cream
- Almond milk yogurt
- Chia seeds
- Ripe avocado

Blending Tips and Tricks

We always want the best-tasting smoothies in the shortest time possible, so a few tips can come in handy to make things easier and speed the process along.

You can use a high-speed electric stand blender, or a jug and an immersion blender to make smoothies. The biggest difference between the two is that a stand blender has a more powerful motor. This allows the stand blender to more easily blend firmer ingredients like cruciferous vegetables, frozen ingredients, and ice cubes.

Load the blender jug with your ingredients in the following order:

1. First, pour in the liquid.

2. Then add soft and small ingredients.

3. Place any greens on top of that.

4. Place vegetables and frozen fruit on top of the greens.

5. Lastly, add any ice cubes you would like to use.

A great tool to purchase, if your stand blender does not have it as an accessory, is a blender tamper. You use the tamper to remove any air pockets that might be in the blender jug and to push the ingredients down onto the blender blades.

Be patient, and do not over blend the ingredients. Remember, the motor and blades will heat up fast, and will start melting the frozen ingredients. Blend in bursts of 30-45 seconds and repeat if necessary.

Depending on the ingredients used for a specific smoothie, you may have to stop the blender, scrape the sides clean, and give it another short burst of blending.

If you use coconut, different types of seeds, oats, or whole nuts, add them to the blender with the liquid. Blend these ingredients and the liquid until you have a creamy paste, for approximately 30 seconds. Then add the rest of the ingredients.

If you are not using a high-speed blender, it works much better if you grate vegetables such as zucchini, beets, and carrots before adding to the blender jug.

Smoothie Recipes

Orange and Mango Recovery Smoothie

This smoothie is sweet, with turmeric that adds anti-inflammatory properties that aid recovery. This recipe is vegan and has no added sugar, and is high in vitamin C and antioxidants. The primary source of protein is protein powder.

Prep Time: 5 minutes

Total Time: 5 minutes

Serving Size: 1

Ingredients

- 1 cup almond milk, unsweetened, or other plant milk of your choice
- 1 cup mango blocks, frozen
- 1 scoop (2 heaping tbsp.) vegan protein powder, vanilla
- ½ banana, frozen
- ½ tsp turmeric (optional, to add anti-inflammatory properties)
- 1 naval orange, frozen, peeled and cut up
- ½ tsp vanilla extract or essence
- 1 tbsp. hemp seeds (optional)

Directions

- Layer all the ingredients into a high-speed blender.
- Blend until completely smooth.

- Pour into a glass and enjoy it.

Green Breakfast Protein Smoothie

This is a good smoothie to start the day with vitamins and minerals, plus healthy fats from hemp hearts and pumpkin seeds. You can add protein powder as an optional extra for an increased protein boost.

To make this smoothie nut-free, substitute the almond milk with oat, coconut, hemp, rice, or soy milk.

Prep Time: 5 minutes

Total Time: 5 minutes

Serving Size: 2 cups (1 large serving)

Ingredients

- 1 ripe frozen banana (can be substituted with 2/3 cup peach chunks)
- 1 cup almond milk, unsweetened, or substitute with milk of personal choice
- ½ cup frozen mango chunks
- 1-2 big handfuls of baby spinach, or destemmed kale

- 2 tbsp. hemp hearts (hemp seeds that have been hulled)

- ¼ cup pepitas (pumpkin seeds)

- ½-1 scoop (1-2 heaped tbsp.) protein powder, vanilla flavor

- ¼ cup water (optional)

Directions

Place all the ingredients into the blender jug and blend until the pepitas are completely blended in and smooth.

This is a large serving, so you can either have it for breakfast, or split it into 2 smaller servings and have the second half as a morning snack.

Cinnamon, Oats, and Apple

If you are an oatmeal lover, this is definitely the smoothie for you. It is suitable for breakfast, a morning snack, or lunch. Oats give a slow release of energy that will last several hours, and the oats and almond butter are your main sources of protein. You can also add hemp hearts for higher protein intake, and the hemp does not affect the taste of the smoothie. For a hefty protein boost, you can add vanilla protein powder as well.

Prep Time: 5 minutes

Total Time: 5 minutes

Serving Size: 1 large serving

Ingredients

- ½ cup oats, rolled
- 1 small-to-medium sliced apple
- ½ tsp ground nutmeg
- ½ tsp cinnamon powder
- ½ cup coconut milk, unsweetened
- 1 tbsp. almond butter
- 2 tbsp. hemp hearts (optional)
- 1 scoop (2 heaping tbsp.) vanilla protein powder (optional)
- ½ cup water, cold
- 3-4 ice cubes

Directions

- Place the water and oats into the blender jug and pulse a few times. Set the jug aside for 2-3 minutes to give the oats time to soften.

- Add the rest of the ingredients to the blender and process for roughly 30 seconds, until the mixture is smooth.

- Pour into a large glass and sprinkle with extra nutmeg and cinnamon as garnish.

- Enjoy immediately.

Acai Berry and Mint

This is a smoothie for literally any time of the day, for breakfast, post-workout, or as a morning snack. Using unflavored protein powder allows the mint and fruit taste to stay in the foreground. Adding ground seeds makes this a thick smoothie with a very good protein supply. The mango and tart cherry puree and acai berry puree can be store-bought in single-serving packets, or you can use your own frozen fruit from your freezer.

Prep Time: 5 minutes

Total Time: 5 minutes

Serving Size: 1 large

Ingredients

- 1 frozen banana, sliced

- 1 orange, fresh (Cara Care, Valencia, and Navel oranges work well)

- ½ cup mango, frozen, or 1 packet tart cherry and mango puree, frozen (3.5 oz.)

- 3.5 oz. of frozen Acai berries, or 1 packet of frozen Acai puree (3.5 oz.)

- 1 tbsp. flax seeds, ground

- 1 tbsp. chia seeds, ground

- 1 scoop (2 heaping tbsp.) protein powder, unflavored

- 2 tbsp. hemp seeds, ground

- ½ cup coconut milk, unsweetened

- 4-5 mint leaves, fresh

Directions

- Place all the ingredients into the blender jug and blend until the mixture is smooth.

- Pour into a large glass and serve immediately, while still cold.

Avocado and Matcha with Vanilla

This smoothie is energizing, and the matcha, which is a form of powdered green tea, has great health properties. This recipe is gluten and soy-free. You can keep this smoothie with just the basic ingredients, or add any of the optional ingredients as preferred.

Prep Time: 5 minutes

Total Time: 5 minutes

Serving Size: 1

Ingredients

- 1 cup almond milk, or milk of personal preference
- ½ avocado
- ½-1 tsp matcha powder (start off with ½ tsp, as it is potent)
- 1 scoop (2 heaping tbsp.) protein powder, vanilla (rice or pea protein works well)
- 2-4 ice cubes
- ½ cup frozen fruit of personal choice (optional)
- 2 tbsp. chia seeds, flax seeds, or pepitas (optional)
- A few dates for sweetness (optional)

- 1-2 tsp maple syrup for extra sweetness (optional)

Directions

- Place all the ingredients into the blender and blend until smooth.

- Serve immediately.

Cranberry, Banana, and Peanut Butter

Cranberries are a winner in any smoothie because they are high in vitamins and antioxidants, and have anti-inflammatory properties as well. The banana and cranberries are sweet, so it is suggested that you use unsweetened ingredients with them. Should you prefer to make it sweeter, use peanut butter with added sugar, and add optional sweetener to the smoothie, such as honey or maple syrup. The source of protein for this smoothie comes from the peanut butter and the protein powder, and gives you roughly 1.2 oz. of protein.

Prep Time: 5 minutes

Total Time: 5 minutes

Serving Size: 1 large portion

Ingredients

- 1 large frozen banana, sliced

- 1 cup coconut milk, unsweetened, or milk of own choice
- 2 tbsp. of peanut butter, unsweetened
- ¼ cup dried cranberries, unsweetened, or sweetened with fruit juice only
- 2 heaping tbsp. unflavored protein powder
- 1 ½ tbsp. ground chia seeds
- 1 tbsp. ground hemp seeds
- 3-4 ice cubes
- Shredded coconut as an optional topping
- Cacao nibs as an optional topping

Directions

- Grind the hemp and chia seeds in a coffee grinder before adding them to the smoothie mixture.
- Place the milk and ground seeds into the blender and pulse until combined.
- Add all the remaining ingredients and blend until the mixture is smooth.

- Pour smoothie into a large glass, add the optional topping if using, and enjoy.

Quinoa with Strawberry and Banana

Quinoa is very high in protein and contains all of the nine essential amino acids that your body needs, and is also high in magnesium and fiber. Chia seeds are the richest plant-based source of Omega 3, and provide more Omega 3 than salmon. Wheat germ adds fiber and vitamin B to the smoothie to make this an all-round protein and vitamin-packed smoothie for any time of the day. You can cook the quinoa beforehand and then measure it out into single portions and freeze it to save time and effort.

Prep Time: 6 minutes

Total Time: 6 minutes

Serving Size: 2 (4 cups)

Ingredients

- ½ cup cooked quinoa, cooled down
- 1 ripe banana, large
- 2 tbsp. honey
- 6 oz Greek yogurt, vanilla

- 1 tbsp. wheat germ
- 1 tbsp. chia seeds
- 2 cups frozen strawberries (if using fresh strawberries, freeze them first)
- 1 ½ cups almond milk, vanilla flavor (or milk of own choice)
- 1 tsp xanthan gum (optional if you prefer a thicker smoothie)
- 1 cup ice cubes

Directions

- Place all the ingredients into a blender jug and blend for roughly 45 seconds, until the mixture is smooth.
- Pour into two large glasses and serve immediately.

Banana, Peach, and Honey

This smoothie is popular with adults and children for breakfast or a snack. The main source of protein is cottage cheese. Unflavored protein powder can be added for an extra super protein boost. The recipe makes 2 large smoothies, or 3 medium-sized ones.

Prep Time: 5 minutes

Total Time: 5 minutes

Serving Size: 2 large smoothies

Ingredients

- 2 ½ cups of peach slices, frozen
- 1 banana, ripe and fresh or frozen
- 1 cup milk (full cream, non-fat, or fat-free,) can be substituted with any plant-based milk
- 1 cup of cottage cheese, preferably cultured
- 2 tbsp. honey (more or less, can be used as per personal preference)

Directions

- Place all the ingredients into the blender and blend until you have a smooth consistency.
- Pour into two large glasses and serve.

Pineapple and Raspberries

This recipe yields 3 cups as a single serving. If you find this too much, you can optionally add in plain cottage cheese and more milk, and then split the smoothie into

2 servings. The source of protein comes from the protein powder, and the cottage cheese if you add that.

Prep Time: 5 minutes

Total Time: 5 minutes

Serving Size: 1 very large serving (3 cups)

Ingredients

- ½ cup frozen or fresh raspberries
- 1 cup frozen pineapple chunks
- 1 cup of unsweetened coconut milk
- ½ tsp Stevia or honey (optional)
- 2 tbsp. vanilla protein powder of your own choice
- ½ cup ice
- ½ cup cultured plain cottage cheese (optional extra)
- ¼ cup extra coconut milk (optional extra if you are adding cottage cheese)
- Shredded coconut, unsweetened, as a topping

Directions

- Place all the ingredients into the jug of a high-speed blender and blend until the mixture has a thick, creamy texture.

- Pour into one very large glass, or into two medium-sized glasses.

- Top with shredded coconut or any other topping of your own choice and serve.

Cantaloupe and Ginger Smoothie

This smoothie recipe focuses mainly on cantaloupe instead of the usual assortment of fruit, nuts, seeds, and vegetables that go into most smoothies. The main source of protein here is from Greek yogurt and cottage cheese. Unflavored protein powder can be added if you need to add extra protein to your diet.

You can turn this smoothie into a smoothie bowl by adding an extra ½ cup of Greek yogurt and topping with toasted coconut, chopped kiwi fruit, and chia seeds.

Prep Time: 7 minutes

Total Time: 7 minutes

Serving Size: 2 cups (2 servings of 1 cup or 1 large serving)

Ingredients

- 2 ½ cups of peeled cantaloupe, cut into blocks
- 1 cup Greek yogurt, plain
- ½ cup cultured cottage cheese
- 1 tsp fresh ginger, peeled and grated
- ½ tsp lime zest, finely grated
- ½ scoop (1 heaping tbsp.) unflavored protein powder (optional)
- 2 tsp honey or maple syrup

Directions

- Pack all the ingredients into the blender and process for about 30-60 seconds, until the mixture is smooth and thick.
- Serve immediately as one large smoothie, or two servings of 1 cup each.

Chapter 8:

7-Day Training Guide Plan

The following is a 7-day training guide to walk you through the first week of calisthenics.

Monday

These exercises are calisthenics building blocks that will help you build strength and endurance. They'll set a basis for performing the more demanding movement in the future. Perform four cycles of the following exercises:

- A plank:
    - Put your hands underneath your shoulders.
    - Ground toes into the floor so that your body is in a neutral position.
    - Hold for 30 seconds.
- Eight squats:

- Stand straight, feet slightly wider than the hips, and point toes outwards.
- Look straight in front of you, with a straightened, but not stiff, neck.
- Raise your arms parallel to the ground with a neutral spine.
- Squat with spine, with the core slightly flexed.
- Push hips back.
- Squat.
- Stand back up in the right position.

- Eight lunges on each leg:
    - Stand tall, with feet aligned with hips.
    - Step forward with one leg.
    - Lower the body until the thigh parallels the floor.
    - Stand back up.

- Eight pushups:
    - On the ground, place hands slightly wider than shoulders.

- Make feet well-balanced.
- Keep spine and core in a neutral position.
- Lift yourself up until your arms are straight.
- Go back down.
- Eight lay-down leg raises:
  - Lie down with your legs extended and arms flat against your body.
  - Join legs together and lift them up.
  - Keep core flat against the floor.
  - Lower back down and repeat.
- 20 mountain climbers on each leg:
  - Position into a plank.
  - Pull one knee into the chest.
  - Straighten the leg out.
  - Repeat.
- Eight pike push-ups:
  - Get in a push-up position.

- Lift your hips and form an upside-down V.

- Bend arms at the elbow until you nearly touch the floor.

- Push yourself up and repeat.

Tuesday: Basic Exercises

Today, you will introduce yourself to more basic calisthenics exercises. These exercises will require a bar for you to hang from. A quality bar will be an investment, but you can find many that are reasonably priced so that you don't have to overspend.

You'll do four cycles of the following exercises:

- Seven close-hand chin-ups:

    - Stand in front of a pull up bar.

    - Grab it with an overhand grip.

    - Lift your body, with hands around a foot apart.

    - Pull yourself up until your chin is above the bar.

- - Return to the starting position and repeat.
- Five pull-ups
- Six dips
  - Stand between parallel bars and jump up while holding onto the bars.
  - Lower your body with arm-bending and dip until your elbows are slightly below the bars.
  - Lift yourself back up.
  - Repeat.
- Fifteen push-ups
- Five leg raises
- Nine jump squats:
  - Stand straight, feet shoulder-width apart.
  - Jump up.
  - Lower the body into the squat position when landing.
  - Repeat.

- 15 Australian pull-ups:
    - Wrap a towel around a door knob on each side of your door.
    - Stand aligned with the door edge, one foot on each side of the door.
    - Squat down while holding onto the towel, with your elbows parallel to the ground.
    - Pull yourself as far back as you can without extending the arms.
    - Pull yourself back towards the door.
    - Repeat.

Wednesday: Rest

Remember how we talked about the importance of active resting? Today, you shouldn't actively exercise, but instead opt-in for up to an hour of light walking in the fresh air, or up to fifteen minutes of light jogging. Remember to adjust your meals to your activity levels! On rest days, you should eat slightly less than when you're working out, but still enough to support muscle recovery.

Thursday

Today, you'll do four cycles of:

- Wide push-ups, 20 repetitions:
    - Position for regular pushups, hands wider than shoulders.
    - Bend elbows outwards.
    - Lift yourself up, pause, then pull yourself down.
- Mountain climbers, 20 of each
- A one-minute wall sit:
    - Stand against the wall with a flat back.
    - Hold feet shoulder-width apart.
    - Bend down with back flat against the wall, until your thighs parallel the ground.
    - Hold the position for 60 seconds.
    - Repeat.
- A one-minute plank

- Clap push-ups, 15 repetitions:
    - Start off by lifting yourself up in a regular push-up position.
    - Propel yourself to lift hands off the ground.
    - Clap once your hands lift off the ground.
    - Return to the starting position.
    - Repeat.
- A half-minute superman hold:
    - Lie down on your stomach.
    - Extend arms and legs.
    - Lift arms and legs up so that your body is in an arched position.
    - Hold for 30 seconds.
    - Return to the starting position.
- Squats, 30 repetitions

Remember to hydrate while exercising!

Friday: Fat Loss

It's time to do a little bit more cardio to get rid of excess fat. Today, you'll do four cycles of:

- A 100-meter run
- Five dips
- Eight push-ups
- Jumping jacks for 45 seconds:
    - Stand straight.
    - Keep your legs together and arms at sides.
    - Jump and spread your legs while lifting arms over the head.
    - Return to the starting position.
    - Repeat for 45 seconds.
- A 15-second plank
- Mountain climbers with alternating knees, 30 repetitions

Saturday: Cardio

Not going to work today? In that case, it's a great time to do some more cardio. It may not be what you hoped for, but remember that cardio exercises benefit your cardiovascular health and endurance of physical stress. Today, you will do:

- Four cycles of 15-second sprints, followed by a 45-second walk

- One cycle of a 30-minute sprint and a 90-second walk

- Four cycles of a 15-second sprint followed by a 45-second walk

- One cycle of a 30-second sprint and a 90-second walk

Now, you will break a sweat—don't doubt it.

Sunday: Rest

Chapter 9:

Calisthenics Workout: Muscle Groups and Body Splits

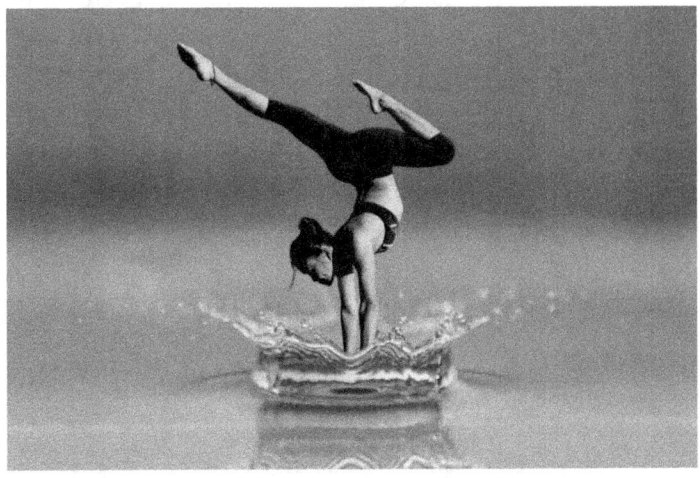

The beauty of calisthenics lies in the fact that it never engages just one single muscle. It always engages one or multiple muscle groups, giving you a gracious, natural form that grows straight out of the natural shapes and forms of your body. In the previous chapter, you learned how to plan and track your progress with calisthenics. Now, the fun begins! In this chapter, you will learn which exercises train specific muscle groups, so that you can choose depending on your personal goals.

While the calisthenics exercises are too numerous to explain in this beginner manual, you can roughly divide them by the muscle groups they activate:

- **Upper body push.** These exercises stimulate the chest, anterior and medial shoulders, and triceps. They are beneficial for stabilizing shoulder positioning when you're performing pushing-away movements. These exercises can be further divided into horizontal and vertical.

- **Upper body pull.** These exercises train your posterior shoulders, biceps, lats, trapezius, and rhomboids muscles. They help you balance shoulder muscles and pull yourself up when exercising.

- **Knee flexion.** These exercises include different variations of squats, and they train muscles involved in squatting, like adductors, quadriceps, glutes, and hip muscles. Training these muscles enables you to squat in the right position.

- **Single leg**. These exercises help you balance your body when standing on one leg. They strengthen your core, adductors, and quadriceps, and improve your coordination and balance.

- **Hip extensions**. Stretching and flexing hip muscles engages the lower back, glutes, and hamstrings. They help you maintain a straight posture and prevent injuries when exercising.

- **Core stabilizers**. These exercises include the famous plank and its many variations. They engage your upper and lower core muscles.

The so-called upper-lower body split is quite popular among calisthenics exercisers. While there are many principles and methods you can use and apply as you advance your training, this method might be the most beginner-friendly, because it's most concise. The upper-lower body split splits your training sessions to target each muscle group at least once during the week. Research shows that exercises using traditional split methods lead to better progress and fewer injuries. However, research also shows that targeting one body part for each day of the week is a less successful method, because the individual body parts get too much resting time.

How Much Should You Exercise?

Optimally, you allow for up to three days for each of the muscle groups to recover. This means that you should target a specific muscle group at least twice a week. The best way to progress is to exercise multiple times each week. Research shows that those who exercise twice a week show better muscle growth than those who exercise only once. If you train twice per week and do it accurately, you should see a 6.8% muscle growth after a couple of weeks (Peterson et al., 2004).

But how many, and which muscle groups should you target each week?

You can successfully add a training session for each muscle group without increasing the number of sessions. Instead, you can do this by focusing on a single muscle group per each training session. If you split to the upper and lower body, this means that one session will be dedicated to the upper body, and another one to the lower body. Still, you should make sure that all of the muscle groups have enough time to recover.

How to Train Different Muscle Groups?

So, how do you do upper-lower body split workouts? The answer is simple. One day of the training is dedicated to upper-body exercises, and the other to the lower body.

- **Upper body exercises** engage chest muscles, upper and middle back, forearm, arm muscles, and shoulders. Exercisers usually have to find a way to incorporate forearm exercises into their body routine, which can be done by adding pull-ups and deadlift exercises.

- **Lower body exercises** engage the muscles in your stomach, lower back, quads, hamstrings, glutes, and calves.

One of the greatest advantages of this exercise model is that it maximizes the gains from engaging individual muscle groups once per week. As you progress with the exercises, you can add more repetitions and sets.

When you engage the muscles of a certain group, they grow in the size of the muscle cells. This is called hypertrophy. Muscle hypertrophy in the upper body is achieved mechanically, by adding physical stress to the muscles, or muscle damage, that stimulates muscles to grow stronger and bigger, and metabolic stress, which happens when chemical products of anaerobic metabolism build-up.

This is important to keep in mind, because targeting muscle size doesn't always improve muscle strength. You'll use different strategies to become bigger and to be physically stronger. You should aim to do exercises that cause hypertrophy if you want to increase the size of your muscles.

The following beginner fundamental exercises engage main muscle groups and enable you to move onto other, more demanding exercises:

- **Push-ups** engage your hands and consist of using your hands to push yourself up and then let down slowly. They engage upper chest muscles, triceps, and shoulders, and stabilize your abs, back, legs, and traps. Aside from the famous handstand, push-up exercises give you stability when lifting heavy objects. They are compound horizontal exercises. A correct push-up is done by letting your chest get as close to the ground as possible. Aside from the mentioned muscles, proper exercise will also engage your upper and lower back.

- **Pull-ups** include compound vertical pulling exercises that are done on a bar, pulling your body upwards. These exercises engage abs, biceps, and shoulders mainly, and other muscle groups, like those in your legs, when you're pulling your body up. Doing these exercises strengthens muscles needed to climb and pull down objects. Aside from being able to maneuver shelf objects with much grace, pull-ups will also help you perform other activities and exercises that demand you to grab, pull, and climb. Beginner pull-ups include leg assisted, half pull-ups, and full pull-ups.

- **Squats** are compound exercises that engage your lower body. A proper squat is done by bending your knees until you touch your hamstrings with your calves. After that, you press back up. These exercises engage your abs, side abs, and lower back, aside from leg muscles. They stabilize your whole body, strengthen your core, and help you stay balanced. Modified versions include assisted half and full squats, half squats, and full squats.

- **Leg raises** strengthen both the front and back core. Exercising them requires lifting the legs until they are parallel with the floor. They mainly target abdominal muscles and improve hip flexion and extension. They also stabilize your legs, making your core strong and creating visible abs.

- **Planks** strengthen your core and train abs while stabilizing muscles. To do a plank properly, you should get into a push-up position with your feet joined together. Your forearms should rest on the ground, and the position should be held for as long as possible. Planking is one of the most demanding exercises, but best known for its results.

- **Dips** are among the most effective and most important calisthenics exercises. They are done using parallel bars. The easy-looking exercise requires you to push your body in while holding onto the bars. To do them correctly, your brachialis should point forward and your elbows should be right next to your body. Your scapula should remain tense and be slightly pressed down, with your neck straight. Your pelvis should be tipped back, and your legs straight to keep your spine straight and stable. This exercise will engage your triceps and strengthen mainly core muscles, but also your thighs.

What is Hypertrophy, and How to Achieve It?

To achieve muscle hypertrophy, you'll need more repetitions than you'd need for muscle strength.

Metabolic stress is mainly triggered by an increase in exercise volume, and it is the main factor that causes hypertrophy. Up to 25% of muscle growth happens because of metabolic stress.

However, simply increasing exercise volume won't be enough for the desired result. Research shows that you should work on each muscle group three times per week. This is a measure best suited for both athletes and nonathletes. More precisely, four sets per muscle group at 60%, one-repetition maximum, will provide the best result, combined with proper intensity and adequate split.

Athletic physique, on the other hand, if you want to maintain or progress, will need a higher volume training, done twice per week. Athletes usually exercise eight sets per each muscle group at 85%. This training regime gives greater volume, and best-optimized hypertrophy.

How to Schedule Your Workout Sessions

But how to schedule your sessions for the best results? Your schedule should be simple and attainable. It should be easy to follow by keeping up a three to four-day exercise schedule. Here's a suggestion for your exercise days:

- Monday and Thursday - upper body exercises
- Tuesday and Friday - lower body exercises
- Wednesday, Saturday, and Sunday - rest days

During the rest days, you should be recovering actively by doing light cardio and other low-intensity activities. For example, you should take light walks or jogs. You can vary this schedule if you want to, to introduce more variety into your routine, or adjust your workout schedule to your weekly schedule. Here are some suggestions for how to vary your three-day routine throughout two weeks:

First week

- Monday and Friday - lower body
- Wednesday -upper body
- Tuesday, Saturday, and Sunday - rest days

Second week

- Monday and Friday - upper body
- Wednesday - lower body
- Tuesday, Saturday, and Sunday - rest days

This schedule will give you similar efficiency to the four-day split, at a lower frequency for different muscle groups. It will work well for those who have a busy schedule and can't find the time to work out four times a week.

How to Include Cardio Exercises

Cardio exercises are usually more popular with people who are after weight loss than muscle and strength building. You should still include cardio training into your routine even if you're not looking to lose weight, because they are good for your cardiovascular health. If you are trying to lose weight, you should keep in mind that strength exercises are often equally or even more effective than cardio.

When you're working with limited time capacity, you should do around twenty minutes of cardio training after each session of strength training. High-intensity intervals will help maximize workout time. You can also add cardio training to everyday activities, like jogging from and back to your home, and whenever the occasion is suitable.

When you start doing your exercises, it's very likely that you'll experience some stress and loss of motivation. However, there are things you can do to prevent and improve this. You should make sure to keep up with your schedule, because results that will show will most certainly help improve your motivation.

How to Exercise Your Core

Core strength will give you not only stability with other exercises, but also joint flexibility and motor control. And, let's face it, everyone wants a tight stomach with prominent chest muscles. While the majority of popular core exercises belong to the intermediate level, there's still plenty for beginners to enjoy. Core exercises strengthen the three important elements of successful calisthenics, which include joint flexibility, motor control, and core strength. Here are some of the beginner-friendly exercises that address all three important aspects:

Core Flexibility

- **Hip rotations**. Start the exercise by lying with bent knees and feet together, with a flat back. Drop both of your legs to one side and hold for up to 30 seconds. Bring legs to the center and move to the other side. Repeat the exercise three times.

- **Lumbar extension.** Lie on your stomach and place your hands underneath your shoulders. Your glutes and pelvis should touch the ground as you push your chest up from the floor. Hold the position up to ten seconds, and repeat up to five times.

- **Hip stretches.** Kneel and step forward with your left leg, so that it's in a lunge position. Tilt your pelvis forward and hold the position for 20 seconds, after which you'll repeat with the other leg. You should do this exercise three times.

Core Strength

- **Leg lowers.** Lie on your back with your legs up at a 90-degree angle. Your back should be flat, not arched, as you lower one of your legs until it touches the ground. Pull the leg back up and repeat with the other leg. You should practice 10 times with each leg, while making sure that your back doesn't arch. Take a minute break after each set.

- **Arabesque.** Stand on one leg and bring the other back. Lower your trunk to parallel the floor, then return to the standing position. Complete two sets of 10 repetitions on each side.

- **Single leg squats**. Stand on a pillow with one leg and lower your body by bending at your knee and hip. Complete two sets of 20 repetitions.

Core Control

- **Arm and leg alterations**. Position yourself into a four-point kneel. Make sure that your lower back is parallel to the floor, and not arched. Lift the opposite arm and leg at the same time and extend them, while making sure that your back and pelvis are aligned. Practice two sets of 20 repetitions.

- **Bridge**. Lie flat with your knees bent. Lift your bottom from the floor by engaging core muscles. Practice two sets of up to 20 repetitions.

Chapter 10:

10 Tips for Making Motivation Last

Now you know what calisthenics is all about, what you need to do to exercise properly, how to eat, when to rest, and all the other essentials. Still, if regular exercise was so easy, the world would be much fitter and leaner, and obesity would've been eradicated. But it's not like that, is it? One of the bigger challenges with calisthenics lies in the fact that it's done independently. There's no one to supervise you and give direction in case you're not exercising correctly.

Why Have You Lost the Motivation to Exercise?

There are several reasons why people lose motivation to learn calisthenics. The first reason is that they repeat the same exercises and routines over and over again, and become bored with it after a while. To a certain degree, this can be due to the lack of knowledge about how to alter exercises to achieve a good result. A repetitive exercise regimen no longer stimulates your body, and so you don't feel like doing it anymore. You stop seeing results and lose your motivation. Another important reason is that exercisers become too focused on targeting the core and forget that, in calisthenics, each exercise serves a purpose, and all of them affect different muscle groups indirectly.

The third reason for the loss of motivation could be that you're over-exercising and not getting enough rest. If training consumes your daily schedule and you get too caught into planning and measuring progress, it becomes an obsession. A sport that once served to deepen your physical awareness and sharpen your skills falls victim to self-policing, so you feel like a prisoner of it in a way. The lack of time to rest and unwind, listen and observe your body, and more importantly, forgetting that calisthenics is more than exercise, kills your motivation.

So, what do you do when you get stuck in a rut? The best way out of it is to reflect on the meaning of calisthenics and its significance for your life and health. This way, you will again find beauty and fun in it. Should the aforementioned happen to you, there are numerous ways to regain your motivation. The following sections will give you some suggestions to regain your motivation and start exercising devotedly once again.

When You Feel Like Giving Up, Remember to...

Start Small

When you're just starting out with calisthenics, it may look as if achieving progress and seeing results is too far away. The beginnings are arguably most difficult. You're just getting used to regular exercise, it's possible that your weight is a point of contempt in your daily life, and you've yet to figure out how to fit exercise into your lifestyle. Although the idea of exercising at home and achieving great results sounds appealing, the lack of knowledge and experience can make you doubt your abilities. With this, you can begin to lose motivation to exercise.

First thing's first, focus on getting into a habit of exercising. You don't have to start with a pitch-perfect routine the very first time. You can start with as little as a 10-minute workout, as long as you start getting used to doing physical activity at that time of the week. You shouldn't think in "all or nothing" mode, but instead do whatever you can of your exercises, even if you feel like you can't push through an entire workout. Because you're starting from scratch, you'll feel all the aches and pains beginners go through before they build the fundamental skills.

Stick to the Basics

There are numerous strategies you can use to keep your motivation high while exercising. However, it's important for you to first know some of the mental principles and training misconceptions. The first is that calisthenics isn't a program for you to build muscle and strength quickly and effortlessly. It will take devotion and time, just like any other program. The only way for you to see quick changes is to follow an expensive program that covers specialized equipment, diet, and supplements. Even with this, chances of failure would be quite high, since it would be up to you to make major changes in your diet and activities.

Focus on Consistency Over Intensity

One of the things to consider is that calisthenics is more than simply an exercise program. It is a lifestyle that demands the following essential principles. The first thing you need to understand is that calisthenics doesn't promise overnight success. It requires devoted exercise, tracking your progress, and using your body weight to the maximum if you want to see results. If you are willing to invest time and put effort into training, you'll eventually witness how much your strength, health, and performance can improve. However, this doesn't happen quickly. Safe to say, it will take a couple of months for you to see the first results. Calisthenics has a long history, and has been used by many historic strongmen to make exceptional achievements.

Remember Why You Started

Calisthenics isn't only about exercise and physical strength. It is also about creating a healthy connection with your body and being willing to invest in yourself so that you grow your potential. It will help you become the best version of yourself, so that you can contribute to the world and to those around you. However, most people who become successful because of calisthenics spend over ten years not only exercising, but studying physical strength and learning about this form of exercise. This way, they were able to build themselves up to the greatest levels of success, and are now able to perform push-ups with one arm, or squats with one leg. However, the road there isn't easy for anyone, and it won't be easy for you.

Don't Take an All-Or-Nothing Approach

The second thing you need to understand is that you have more strength than you think. Most people tend to underestimate their capacities and overestimate limitations. Nowadays, people want to see instant success, and feel like they're not capable enough if what they do doesn't show results right away. As with many other things in life, this approach won't help with calisthenics. You simply need to give it time. You'll need to develop devotion and mental toughness going forward, because learning and patience, aside from regular training, are all you need to get where you want to be.

Stick to the Basics

Even reaching the fundamental goals might test your patience and motivation, and there's nothing wrong with that. Keep in mind that you're neither the first nor the last person to doubt their abilities at the very beginning. If you want to succeed, you need to decide that you will push through obstacles and limitations and stay focused on following through with your plan, more than you'll be paying attention to the results you're trying to see. Calisthenics will require a lot of hard work, and it should, because you'll learn devotion and discipline that will transfer onto other areas of your life.

Remind Yourself What's at Stake

You will often find yourself wanting to quit. Whenever you start thinking about giving up, you should think about the health benefits of doing exercise, even if the desired results fail to show. Even if you're exercising and not getting the results you want, you will still be doing better compared to not exercising at all. If you get stuck and start to feel like you want to switch onto another program, focus on the fact that you will most likely have to commit to going to the gym or buying equipment before you can even start, let alone before you see results.

Every workout you do, regardless of how you feel, just for the sheer discipline, strengthens your body and your mind. People who have anxiety or stress-related health issues often find it difficult to perform daily tasks without getting upset at every little unpleasantness, and it is that growing sensitivity that only worsens your health issues. The more you face this overwhelming feeling of not wanting to exercise and just leap into your workout instead, the more you will develop the skills to cope with and overcome other challenges and unpleasantness in life.

Make it Fun!

Another important thing to think about is making your workouts fun. You will most definitely lose your motivation if you only focus on the number of repetitions. There are ways for you to have fun while exercising. If you find yourself bored by doing exercises or they feel too difficult, you can play some music or listen to an e-book. Regardless of your goals, you should have an action plan when you start exercising. Your exercise plan will prevent you from being bored or confused because you don't know how to exercise, or which exercises to use. Having a clear, progressive plan will tell you exactly what to do to see progress. Making your exercise plan is a great first step, but actually following through with it is a different story.

You'll need to develop strategies to fight off sluggishness, stress, tiredness, or boredom before and while working out. Aside from creating an interesting setting for exercise, you should also make sure that you're well-rested and have properly eaten.

Aside from this, tracking your progress will boost your motivation as well. In the next chapter, we'll talk about the importance of keeping track of how many exercises you've done, the repetitions, difficulty, weight loss, and the visible changes in your physique. All of these activities will have a beneficial impact on your motivation as well. You will be able to see how far you've come. Most importantly, you'll be able to tell how exercises that once posed a great challenge have now become easy, and you've moved on to greater challenges. Aside from this, measuring your progress will help you remember just how many new things you learned to do, despite having started with zero knowledge and skill.

This way, whenever you get stuck again and start to feel like you've encountered a challenge you won't be able to overcome, you will look in your workout log and remember which approaches and strategies you used to overcome previous challenges. You will understand which areas you need to improve before moving forward.

Aside from this, you should also be aware of the fact that success is a momentary experience. You are becoming more successful, stronger, fitter, and leaner with each new workout. Knowing what you want to achieve with calisthenics and keeping that image in your mind will keep you going when you get stuck. This way, you will gradually progress day after day.

Last but not least, make sure to have some versatility in your exercising so that it's fun. You should shuffle and change up exercises to add variety and boost muscle strength and endurance. You can do this by changing the order of your exercises, changing the range of repetitions, switching volume, doing variations of different exercises, setting medium goals or milestones, changing the frequency of your training, adding cardio, flexibility, and mobility exercises, training other sports you like, or boosting repetitions.

How to Avoid Future Mistakes

Ultimately, you will regain your motivation if you manage to figure out what went wrong with your training and commit to doing things differently in the future. Tracing your footsteps and realizing where you made a mistake could be useful to prevent future failures. Ask yourself if you made some of the following mistakes:

Hating on Fat

If one of your goals was to lose weight, you could've made the mistake of thinking that all fat is your enemy. Fat loss is essential to gain visible muscle, but you will still need enough body fat to keep your body building strong muscles. Fat is an energy reserve, and although you shouldn't have too much of it, you mustn't become fat-depleted either.

Poor Diet and Cardio Optimization

If the beginning of your journey was marked by the difficulty to control eating and engage in cardio, the initial results and improvement could have driven you to over-exercise while eating too little. This loss of balance in diet and exercise may not only slow down your metabolism, but also cause psychological stress and mental tiredness, aside from physical. So, ask yourself, is it possible that you haven't been eating enough for the amount of exercise you want to do? If needed, increase your meal sizes, and the energy replenishment should, and most likely will, result in a better mood to exercise.

Focused on Result, Not the Process

The first thing one learns about calisthenics, and the thing that is easiest to forget, is that its primary goal is to improve your health and physical skills, not necessarily your looks. If you forget this, chances are that you may over train the exercises that produced the most visible results, and forget about the rest of them. To avoid this, always focus on the process of exercise, and on how you want to exceed your body's limitations with physical movement. This way, your choice of exercise will be different, and better adjusted to the needs and possibilities of your body. They will stimulate both body and mind, so you'll never get tired of them.

Chapter 11:

How to Track Your Progress

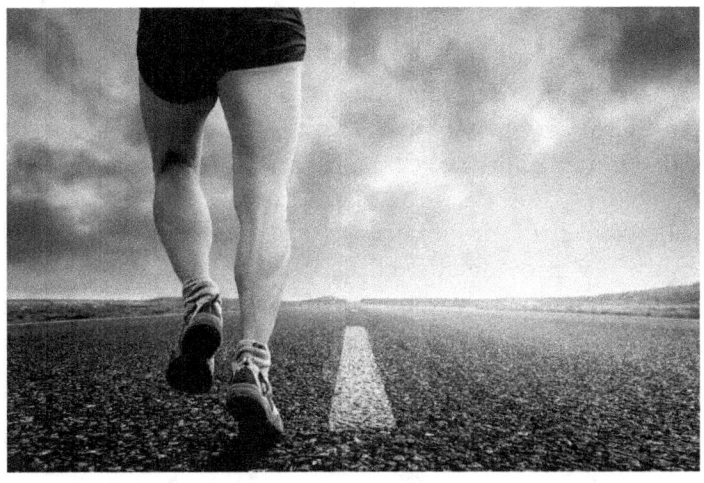

All beginnings are difficult, and doubting whether or not the exercise gives results can make you doubt whether it's worth doing at all. On the other hand, those who are passionate about exercise and physical activity might enjoy it too much, and eventually burn out. How to prevent this? The answer is by keeping track of your progress.

Intuitive vs Planned Training

Should you exercise based on your intuition, or should you develop an exercise program? Some people prefer to follow the wills of their body and do exercises that feel most comfortable, relying on their intuition to tell them what type of movement their body needs. There's logic to that, of course, and the school of intuitive fitness is gaining traction as much as other exercise programs do. Oftentimes, and for certain people, measuring progress is a challenge. Whether because of health limitations or personal circumstances, some just can't commit to a schedule or prioritize their training. Nothing wrong with that, unless your intention is to pursue a skill and make visible progress.

The so-called "autoregulatory training" relies on your body to provide direction for how you shoulder exercises, which exercises to do, and for how long. It relies on "biofeedback evaluation" for the choice of number of sets, repetitions, and types of exercises. Of course, this type of training doesn't guarantee a certain result.

Intuitive training might be wise from time to time, or used with other activities that are more a hobby than they are expected to produce results. If you have a particular goal with calisthenics, and you have an intention to achieve a certain result, then keeping track of your progress is a must. Training without tracking progress keeps you from tracking your goals and noting whether or not you're advancing in the desired direction, and at the desired pace. If you keep track of your exercise, you'll know how many of which exercise you did in your workout sessions, which is especially important when you're aiming to increase training intensity.

Planned training begins with evaluating your starting point and informing yourself of the amount of progress you can achieve given your training background, lifestyle, and health situation. Aside from this, planning helps you build a habit to exercise. If you haven't exercised regularly, making a commitment to work out might be challenging. Planning helps you make physical activity a part of your daily life, and it helps you develop a realistic perspective and expectations for your progress. Planning also helps you keep track of how far you've come, compare current progress with your long-term goal, and pay attention to whether or not your time is spent doing exercises that bring progress.

Writing down your workouts helps track how much you should increase the difficulty of an exercise to progress. After you've spent some time tracking progress, for example after six months, you'll be able to see how close you are to your goal, which mistakes you made, how much you've effectively exercised, and how attainable your goal is. This will help you make better decisions regarding training and bring you closer to your goal.

Tracking your progress will also help you feel more accomplished and boost your motivation to move further. This will assure you that you're investing time and effort wisely, and be satisfied that you're taking enough time to train.

How to Plan Your Calisthenics Training

As a beginner, it's best for you to make a 6-month plan for learning calisthenics. A good plan will contain the workout routines that will serve to produce weight loss or build the amount of muscles you want. Aside from that, it will also include life lessons that you want to learn, and the way in which you will start as a beginner. You'll start making your workout plan by determining how many of each exercise you want to be able to do in six months. However, you will plan for setbacks and failures as well. What if it turns out that your evaluation was wrong, and you don't master the skills you thought you would? In that case, you should plan for so-called regressions, which means using easier modifications of chosen exercises that are a better fit for your body.

Your plan will also determine the types of exercises you should do to increase pulling strength, pushing strength, lower body, and core. After that, you should make a workout plan for one month, and then a weekly plan (which will be given in this book) to follow. Finally, you'll plan progressions, and decide which advanced exercises you'll focus on when increasing the difficulty and volume of training. When you're planning ahead, there's a good chance that you won't make accurate evaluations. That will most likely happen if you plan on your own. But, if you consult a calisthenics expert, they will give experienced advice for what kind of expectations you can set for yourself.

Here's a short example of a six-month plan you can use when planning your training:

- **Basics**. Which warm-up exercises do you want to use, and for how many repetitions? Account for making up to a minute-long break between exercises. Start by mapping out your ability to do five of each: squats, dips, shoulder-width chin-ups, knee raises, and push-ups. If you can't meet these beginner demands just yet, give yourself more time to practice said exercises, and then move to progressions intended for the first month.

- **First month (weeks 1-4)**. At the end of your first month of exercise, you should be able to do ten squats, five push-ups and shoulder chin ups, eight knee raises and chair dips, and at least a minute-long rope jump. A monthly plan should include three workout days, and four (active) rest days.

- **Second month (weeks 5-8)**. By the time you've completed eight weeks of exercise, you should be able to do at least five L-sit chin-ups and decline push-ups, eight dips and hanging leg raises, twelve lunges, and at least three minutes of running. As you can see, these exercises are different compared to the first month, as diversity is important to avoid boredom.

- **Third month (weeks 9-12)**. If you achieved your previous goal, you're now entering the intermediate level. By the end of your twelfth week, you should be able to do five high chest pull ups and straight-on-bar dips, eight leg raises and decline push-ups, twelve calf raises on each leg, and duck-walk for thirty seconds.

- **Fourth month (weeks 13-16)**. You should set your mind to doing ten horizontal jumps, eight pike push-ups and Australian pull-ups, six straight bar dips, five jump muscle ups, and a minute of mountain climbers.

- **Fifth month (weeks 14-17)**. You are approaching your six-month goal! By the end of week 17 of your program, you should set your mind to doing a half-minute frog stand, a minute-long rope jump, three muscle-ups, skin the cats, and chin-above-bars, and 10 vertical jumps.

- **Sixth month (weeks 18-21)**. After six months of training, you should manage four muscle ups, fifteen dips and pushups, and ten jumping squats on a three-minute limit.

The 7-day training guide given in this book will be adjusted for beginners, but feel free to adjust it to your abilities. Keep in mind that practicing below your ability won't show results, and trying to do exercises that are too difficult could result in overstrain and injury.

How to Track Your Progress

Here's what you should track regarding your progress in calisthenics:

- Entire workout sessions and exercises with date, and start and finish time
- Number of sets and repetitions
- Rest and recovery periods and practices
- Warm-ups
- Cool-downs

You can also rate your degree of discomfort, forms you achieved, and levels of exhaustion on a scale from one to 10. When it comes to doing exercises, your pain should be below grade three. If it exceeds it, you should switch to a different variation or better observe your form.

When it comes to your form, you should be tracking how accurately you performed an exercise. Your form score should be at least a nine.

These scores will help you decide how to repeat each consecutive workout or set. When it comes to more difficult exercises, you should pay better attention to the form. The proper form protects against injury, and doing more difficult exercises with an improper form increases your risk from injury. If you can't perform at a score of at least nine, you should consider doing an easier variation of the exercise.

With proper tracking, you should be able to reflect on the quality of your training accurately and note what you can do differently with the next workout to improve. Your exhaustion levels can vary with your exercise program and each individual exercise. However, your exhaustion level should still be between six and eight. Aside from this, you can also keep track of how you feel and what you think about while exercising, and your ideas and suggestions for future workouts.

At the very least, you should keep a workout journal. You can take notes during the workout to trace your performance. Don't lose count of repetitions, and you can also write down your exercise scores. It's also wise to lay out your workout structure before you start. This way, you can just add multiple sessions without putting too much thought into the process.

After the workout, you can write down the notes and observations that you weren't able to write during exercise. You can also write down your notes after the exercise, but the sooner the better. If you wait too long after you've exercised, you can forget some of the important details.

If you don't feel like keeping a journal, there are many other ways for you to track your progress. You can write in a regular notebook that you can take with you anytime you're working out, or you can write down your notes on your phone or tablet. You can also use tracking on your computer to log your exercises. However, make sure that logging doesn't take up too much time, or distract you from exercising. Experienced exercisers find simple notebooks to be the best option because they are the least distracting.

Optionally, you can get a workout log. This log is essentially a notebook, with a template designed to log exercises and other relevant items.

Aside from logging, there are a couple of other ways to keep track of your performance and progress. You can take your measurements if you're pursuing muscle gain or weight loss. You should do this weekly or monthly by measuring the circumference of your arms, waist, forearms, neck, and other parts of the body. You can also take pictures and observe your transformation over the years. You should take three monthly pictures, front, rear, and back. Your muscles shouldn't be flexed or pumped on these images, but natural and taken in natural light.

You can also keep track of your weight by measuring it on a scale. Depending on your goals, you can also do this as often as daily, or once a month. Your body-fat composition is another important item to measure. If you want your body fat to reduce, you should get a body-fat caliper and document your percentages on a monthly or weekly basis.

How to Evaluate Your Progress with Calisthenics

Ultimately, you should work out a method for measuring your progress. So, which metrics should you use with bodyweight training? There are three types of measurements to evaluate your improvement:

- **Exercise progress.** You should track your total training volume, or number of repetitions done per training session, how much time it takes to perform the same number of repetitions, and the quality and accuracy of your exercises (how well you're aligned, how you maintain form, how difficult it is to make repetitions, and how slowly you can do a movement).

- **Physique progress**. Here, you will track and evaluate how much your progress is notable in your shape and size. In calisthenics, physique improves with other improvements of skill, so it is a side-effect in a way. You can measure your weight and follow with body circumference measurements to see how much regular exercise affects your physique.

- **Performance progress**. Lastly, you can track how much your speed, strength, and other physical abilities have improved since you started training. If you're training calisthenics to improve not only looks, but also health and productivity, you can note your energy levels, stress resilience, and how exercise affects your emotional and psychological stability. These can be valuable in case visible changes fail to show significantly, because they remind you of how the quality of your life improved with regular exercise.

Chapter 12:

11 Biggest Myths About Calisthenics

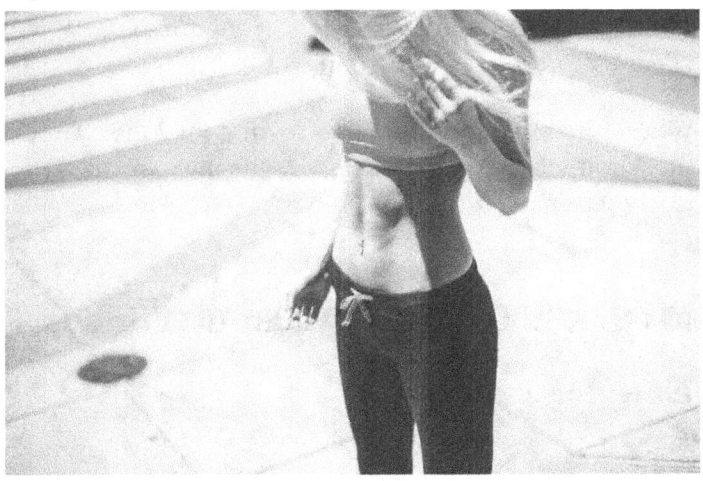

There are so many myths and misconceptions out there, and especially on the internet, that it will make your head spin. The biggest problem with these myths is that they can cause harm and frustration, especially for people starting out on the journey of getting their bodies into shape.

It is important to go through all these myths and misconceptions, as many of them are so ingrained in the fitness scene that they are accepted as truth. The last thing any person starting out with calisthenics needs is to have their progress sabotaged and their fitness goals delayed. The other reason to debunk myths is to not fall into the trap when well-meaning friends and family give advice based on misconceptions and myths. This can easily lead to strained relationships, whereas when you are armed with facts, you can politely and graciously defuse any situation.

Where there is more than one myth concerning a topic or action, they are listed under one heading for easy reference and clarity.

Myth #1: The Best Workout Time is Early Morning

Early mornings are great for doing your daily workout, and if you are a morning person, it is the perfect way to start your day. You also do not have to then make time during your day for your workout, because it is all done with. There is, however, not really a difference whether you prefer to do your workout first thing in the morning or later during the day, at a time more suitable to your personal schedule.

According to a 2019 study, there is no difference in the quality of a workout done first thing in the morning or, for instance, between 1 p.m. and 4 p.m. in the afternoon (Youngstedt, Elliott, & Kripke, 2019). The best time depends on each individual and their daily schedule.

Always Do Cardio First

Many people prefer to do the cardio portion of their exercise at the beginning of their workout so that they can concentrate on other aspects of their session. Cardio exercises draw heavily on your body's glycogen stores within your muscles, whereas other forms of exercise do not. Doing cardio first, in reality, leaves your body with a shortage of glycogen for the rest of your training session. Your weight and strength training will be of poor quality, so switching to doing cardio at the end of your workout gives you a better and more effective workout overall.

Minimum of 20 Minutes Cardio

Often, people fixate on cardio and swear by the 20-minute minimum cardio rule. It is not the time factor in cardio, but instead the intensity of training. You can pack a serious cardio workout into doing high-intensity interval training for a much shorter period. High-intensity interval training is a double plus, as it keeps burning calories once you have completed the workout session.

Another great option to look into for your calisthenics cardio workout is Tabatha training. Tabatha is a form of HIIT, but it takes it to the next level and packs a punch into 4-minute routines that are simply incredible. So, there is no rule that says you must do 20 minutes of cardio for it to be beneficial for you.

More Cardio, More Weight Loss

The idea behind this misconception is that the more cardio you do, the better chance you have of shedding those extra pounds. We are all aware that to lose weight, you must create a calorie deficit, and cardio does contribute to that on a day-to-day basis. However, that is not the smart way to go about losing weight. The smart way is to combine the following things:

Lean muscle mass burns calories while your body is at rest. To create this effect, you need to combine strength training with high-intensity cardio routines.

All your efforts need a solid foundation of a good nutrition plan based on your personal needs.

Cardio Machines Record Calories Burnt Accurately

If you use an elliptical trainer or a treadmill, you should not take the calories burnt display at face value. According to a 2018 study, these machines have a tendency to overestimate the calories burnt per 30-minute workout by at least 100 calories (Glave et al., 2018). This lulls you into a false sense of security, and over time the discrepancy can be quite significant.

Myth # 2: Crunches and Sit-Ups Equal 6-Pack Abs

All ab exercises are great for building and strengthening the muscles of your core. That said, sit-ups and crunches do not automatically give you those sought after 6-pack abs. You have to have a decent eating plan to back up your exercises. You cannot follow a diet high in calories and unhealthy fats if you wish to achieve that ripped look. A thick abdominal subcutaneous layer of fat will hide the tendinous inscriptions completely. Crunches and doing sit-ups alone are not going to work, and even if you can deadlift a significant amount, you need to eat a balanced diet as well.

Myth # 3: Crunches for Core Strength

Crunches are not the beginning and end of core strengthening exercises. Instead of focusing solely on crunches, concentrate on multi-muscle exercises that target all the areas of your core, and not only one.

Fat Is Able to Become Muscle, and Vice Versa

Nobody really knows where this myth started, but muscle tissue and fat are definitely two very different things. Yes, you can lose muscle and gain fat tissue, just as you can build muscle and lose fat. However, there is no magical process that turns the one into the other.

Muscle Loss Starts After 7 Days of Being Inactive

When you have recently started a workout routine and you take a week off, the progress you have gained will be eradicated in a short time. This is logical. It is very different, however, if you have an established workout routine and have been doing it for several months. A study done in 2007 with athletes showed that their performance showed very little deterioration for a period of up to 3 weeks of being inactive (McMaster et. al., 2013).

Myth #4: No Pain, No Gain

Pain warns the body that something is wrong, so the myth that your workout was not effective unless you are sore afterward is a total misconception. Yes, muscle stiffness can be felt after an intense workout, but sharp or intense pain means to stop whatever you are doing and consult your healthcare provider.

Should you feel discomfort and muscle aches after a workout, you should refuel your body, stay hydrated, and rest to allow your body to recover.

Myth #5: Running Is Better Than Walking

This is a misconception that often causes confusion. Running and walking target the exact same groups of muscles, and the only difference is the intensity. The health results of walking and running are the same when you look at the energy expended and calories burnt. The difference is that it takes twice the amount of time for walking to achieve what running does.

So it really is up to the individual whether you want to run, for instance, for 15 minutes, or have a brisk walk for 30 minutes. The only real difference is the time allocated to this activity. Often, a brisk walk with a loved one or a friend has many social and interactive benefits as well.

Myth #6: Sports Drinks Are Healthy

Hydrating after a workout is a great idea, but downing a sports drink is not the greatest idea. Sports drinks are loaded with lots of sugar, and the sugarless ones are loaded with artificial sweeteners. You are basically loading up on unnecessary sugar, sodium, and carbs.

Myth #7: Treadmills and Running Outdoors Are Equal

Running outdoors is different as you encounter uneven terrain, run up and down hills, and encounter wind. This means your body uses more energy than when you run on a treadmill inside a gym or at home. You will burn approximately 10% more calories running outdoors than over the same distance running on a treadmill.

Myth #8: Exercise Makes You Hungry

People often confuse their body signals, especially when they have worked out. They need liquid, and confuse it for hunger. Another reason why people think they are ravenous after a workout is that their sugar levels drop. Your body signals your brain about the drop in blood sugar, and we associate this with hunger.

There are also countless conflicting myths about working out and when you should or should not eat.

Never Do Workouts on an Empty Stomach

There are absolutely no scientific or medical facts to support the misconception that you must eat before you start your workout.

Myth #9: Toning My Muscles Is All I Need to Do

Your muscles are actually well toned, as you use them all the time in everything that you do. You don't see the muscles because they are covered by a layer of fat. The problem lies with your diet. Once you start on a balanced diet, you can use workouts to boost your calorie consumption. Soon, those muscles you want to tone will no longer be hidden under a layer of fat.

Myth #10: Men and Women Cannot Do the Same Workouts

It is a total myth that men and women need different exercise routines. Men and women are the same species and have the same physical design. The difference lies in the fact that men carry much higher levels of testosterone than women. This gives men a strength advantage, but there is no reason why men and women cannot do the same workouts.

Women Should Lift Lighter and Do More Reps

This myth is kept alive because in general, women worry about how lifting weights will affect them, and that it will make them bulk up. Logically, though, women don't lift the same weight as men because of their lower testosterone levels. This also means they do not bulk up in the same way that men do, and women have no need to compensate for this by doing more repetitions.

Men and women should do weight lifting workouts that challenge them, but not overtax or injure them without taking myths to mind.

Yoga Is Not Proper Exercise

The misconception that yoga is not a proper workout and is all about gentle routines with stretching is perpetuated by people who have never taken any yoga classes. The media also portrays yoga as this spiritual and gentle activity. Yes, there are gentle yoga routines, but there are many intense and rigorous routines, for example, power Vinyasa and Bikram yoga. Yoga takes dedication and working out regularly.

Myth #11: Stretching Is a Must to Prevent Injuries

Everyone has heard this at some time during their lives, that you must do stretching exercises before you start your workout, and the dire warnings that you will injure yourself if you don't. Numerous studies over the past decades have found absolutely no proof that doing static stretches before a workout in any way reduces any form of injuries related to exercise.

Yes, it is true that you should not just jump into your calisthenics workout routine without preparation, but you do not have to do stretches. What you need to do is warm-up exercises for about 5-15 minutes, to increase the blood flow to your muscles and loosen the tendons. This is the way to lower the risk of injury during any workout.

Conclusion

Congratulations! You know the basics of calisthenics, and have a good idea of how you can create your exercising plan and start transforming your life, health, and body right now.

The goal of this book was to introduce you to the basics of calisthenics. First, you learned that calisthenics is different from your usual gym workout program. You learned that it is a form of exercise that improves health and beauty most naturally, simply by using the weight of your body and the force of its movement. As you learned, the nature of exercises in calisthenics is such that they don't require lifting weights, only light tools such as bars, rings, bands, and others. You also learned that calisthenics carries a low risk of injury, and that is because your body won't allow you to make movements that are beyond its capabilities. As such, calisthenics is much safer for you and far more effective compared to other forms of exercise.

After that, you learned about the numerous benefits of calisthenics. You first learned that the main benefit of calisthenics comes from the body's own need to move. Our movements are complex and affect both our bodies and minds. You learned that calisthenics utilizes these movements strategically to activate muscles of the entire body in a natural way that grows your muscles and physical strength. As you learned, the lack of movement may cause physical weakness and chronic pains, and calisthenics is a great way to prevent this. You learned that you benefit from calisthenics in numerous physical and mental ways, from losing weight and growing muscles, to regaining emotional and mental balance, regaining healthy sleep, and building discipline, self-responsibility, and accountability. All of these traits, as you learned, will quickly and easily transfer to other areas of your life, affecting not only your fitness and physical ability. They will affect your work and relationships as well, because you'll have strengthened your self-esteem, become a sharper thinker, faster both with work and on your feet, and in better control of your feelings and impulses.

You also learned that to start with calisthenics properly, you need to do it slowly and methodically. You learned that you must start from the simplest exercises and move your way up. You learned that there is no use in comparing yourself to others because your body is one and only. It has its unique abilities, features, and needs. More importantly, you learned that you will do better with calisthenics if you focus more on the process of exercise and enjoy movement, rather than waiting to see the result. As you learned, this type of natural movement deepens your bond with your body and awakens your bodily awareness. The more you exercise, the better you'll recognize the true needs of your body.

As you learned, there's always a risk from injury in sports, even if you practice calisthenics. You learned that there is a risk from overtraining, and that skipping your rest days can not only slow down your progress, but also lead to overtraining syndrome. As you learned, pushing yourself too hard may easily result in temporarily losing the ability to exercise and diminishing the progress made so far.

After that, you learned how exactly calisthenics trains your body. You learned that the three most important principles include the SAID principle, overloading, and progressive overloading. These principles explain that growth of your muscles happens when you add stress or strain that's greater than the level you're used to. When you increase activity levels and load, your entire body, from your brain to the nerves and muscles, adjusts to respond to that stress. That's how the body becomes stronger. You learned that progressive overloading, or increasing the intensity and volume of your exercises once you conquer one level, secures long-term growth and progress.

If you read those sections carefully, you probably came to understand why accurate, well-measured exercises are so important to target muscles by groups and strengthen those you wish. You learned that too little resistance doesn't produce results, and too much leads to burning out. So, what does one do to secure long-term healthy exercise?

The answer is: rest and recover. Upon learning how calisthenics exercises look and which movements to do to target desired upper and lower body muscles, you learned about the enormous importance of rest and recovery. You learned that your muscles don't grow while you exercise, but afterward. You learned that, while you exercise, you cause tiny tears in muscle and ligament tissue. After exercise, rest is vital to allow the body to grow that tissue and fill the micro-tears, hence creating more muscle tissue. You also learned that rest and recovery are vital for the health of your joints and ligaments. You learned that the organs that connect your muscles and tie them to the bones are less supplied with blood, so they need more time to heal compared to muscles.

As you learned, diet and lifestyle play an enormous role in succeeding with calisthenics. You learned that the diet provides fuel for your muscles to grow, and that you need a healthy eating regimen regardless of whether or not you're trying to lose weight. You learned that there's more to your diet than calories. How much protein, carbs, and fat you eat greatly affects how effectively you will learn new skills, and how well your muscles will grow. You learned that both too little and too much of macronutrients gets in the way of healthy exercise. Insufficiency will prevent muscle growth, and too much will deplete fat loss. You learned that you need to balance your macronutrients well if you want to support and stimulate the progressive growth of your muscles and the development of skills.

You learned that eating healthy for the sake of your calisthenics training isn't at all difficult, or expensive. You learned that you only need clean and lean meats, vegetables, fruits, dairy, eggs, nuts and wheat, and legumes, and that you can have them in the amounts that match your exercise goal. You learned that only

200 calories can make a difference between fat gain and fat loss, meaning that adjusting your diet to your goals is much easier than you think.

In this book, you also learned about the importance of defining your goals and planning your exercises and progress. You learned that you need to establish whether your main goal is to lose weight, build muscle, or gain skills. While the chances are that you'll eventually do all three, your primary focus determines your exercise schedule. Those who target weight loss will do more cardio than those going after strength, for example.

Aside from having a clear goal, you also learned how important it is to have an exercise plan based on your goals. You learned that your exercise plan should consist of the types, number, and volume of advanced exercises and abilities you want to achieve for six months. But, as you learned, tracking your progress is vital to know whether you've completed your goals. You learned that you can simply track your progress by writing down how many repetitions you're able to do, how difficult they feel, whether you feel any pain, and how your body has changed during the process.

In this book, you also got a week's-worth of calisthenics exercises to get you going. We focused on the exercises that have proven to be most effective for beginners, and to introduce enough versatility for different types of people to enjoy. You also learned what other exercises you can use to target the muscles of the upper and lower body, and how to exercise and target your goal. With the given exercises, you can now begin the exercises and set your own goals based on what you perceive to need improving.

In terms of improvement, you learned that the lack of flexibility and mobility can get in the way of progress as well. You learned that your tendons, joints, and ligaments can get depleted of blood due to lack of mobility or too much strain. To prevent this, you learned that you need to do flexibility and mobility exercises regularly. You also learned that you need to constantly work on the so-called overhead mobility. You learned that your shoulders can become stiff for numerous reasons, and exercising overhead mobility guarantees that you'll be well-coordinated and strong enough to perform more demanding, advanced exercises.

Finally, you learned about the importance of motivation for exercise. You learned that you may hit a plateau for numerous reasons. It can happen because you followed a too repetitive exercise schedule, because you over trained, because you haven't paid attention to your diet, or because you didn't have enough rest. Either way, you can find yourself stuck, bored, and without the motivation to move forward. As you learned, the solution for this lies in reminding yourself of why you began training calisthenics in the first place, and looking into your unique strengths and needs to find out what's the best way forward. You also learned that there's no need to compare yourself to others. You learned that everyone progresses at their own pace and that your journey is yours alone. You learned that you can bounce back by re-evaluating why you fell in love with calisthenics in the first place, what you wanted to achieve, and also how you might have done things wrong.

You learned that long-term motivation requires finding out where you made a mistake so that you can prevent that mistake from happening in the future. Finally, you learned that there are many misconceptions about calisthenics. You learned that both men and women can do the same exercises, that yoga can be as effective an exercise as all others, that cardio exercises don't always guarantee weight loss, and that you're best off exercising in the fresh air whenever you can.

We want to leave you with a final message to never forget what calisthenics is all about: the harmony between your body and its need for movement. Remember that the best results will come when you focus on your body's natural need to push itself harder, to stretch, pull, and stimulate its tissues. By doing so, you won't worry about your weight or the looks of your abs. You will progress to an amazing level of physical ability, have superb mental and emotional health, and prominent muscles to serve as a cherry on top of the cake.

References

Basso-Vanelli, R. P., Di Lorenzo, V. A. P., Labadessa, I. G., Regueiro, E. M., Jamami, M., Gomes, E. L., & Costa, D. (2016). Effects of inspiratory muscle training and calisthenics-and-breathing exercises in COPD with and without respiratory muscle weakness. *Respiratory care*, 61(1), 50-60.

Beecher, C. E. (1867). Physiology and Calisthenics: For Schools and Families. *Harper*.

Flood, J. E., & Rolls, B. J. (2007). Soup preloads in a variety of forms reduce meal energy intake. *Appetite*, 49(3), 626-634. https://doi.org/10.1016/j.appet.2007.04.002

Gist, N. H., Freese, E. C., Ryan, T. E., & Cureton, K. J. (2015). Effects of low-volume, high-intensity whole-body calisthenics on army ROTC cadets. *Military medicine*, 180(5), 492-498. https://doi.org/10.7205/MILMED-D-14-00277

Glave, A. P., Didier, J. J., & Wagner, M. C. (2018). Calorie expenditure estimation differences between an elliptical machine and indirect calorimetry. *Exercise Medicine*. https://doi.org/10.26644/em.2018.008

McMaster, D. T., Gill, N., Cronin, J., & McGuigan, M. (2013). The development, retention and decay rates of strength and power in elite rugby union, rugby league and American football. *Sports Medicine*, 43(5), 367-384. https://doi.org/10.1007/s40279-013-0031-3

Peterson, M. D., Rhea, M. R., & Alvar, B. A. (2004). Maximizing strength development in athletes: a meta-analysis to determine the dose-response relationship. *The Journal of Strength & Conditioning Research*, 18(2), 377-382. https://doi.org/10.1519/R-12842.1

Thomas, E., Bianco, A., Mancuso, E. P., Patti, A., Tabacchi, G., Paoli, A., ... & Palma, A. (2017). The effects of a calisthenics training intervention on posture, strength and body composition. *Isokinetics and exercise science*, 25(3), 215-222.

Youngstedt, S. D., Elliott, J. A., & Kripke, D. F. (2019). Human circadian phase-response curves for exercise. *The Journal of Physiology*. https://doi.org/10.1113/JP276943

www.ingramcontent.com/pod-product-compliance
Lightning Source LLC
Chambersburg PA
CBHW072153100526
44589CB00015B/2217